Voice Therapy
for Adolescents

Voice Therapy
for Adolescents

By

Moya L. Andrews, Ed.D.
Professor
Department of Speech and Hearing Sciences
Indiana University
Bloomington, Indiana

Anne C. Summers, M.S.
Speech Pathologist
Monroe County Community School Corporation
Bloomington, Indiana

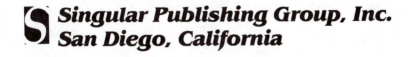
Singular Publishing Group, Inc.
San Diego, California

Singular Publishing Group, Inc.
4284 41st Street
San Diego, CA 92105

Library of Congress Cataloging in Publication Data
Main entry under title:

Andrews, Moya L.
  Voice therapy for adolescents.

  "A College-Hill publication."
  Bibliography: p. 123
  Includes index.
  1. Voice disorders in youth—Treatment. I. Summers,
Anne C., 1941-   II. Title. [DNLM: 1. Voice
Disorders—in adolescence. 2. Voice Disorders—
therapy. WM 475 A568v]
RF511.Y68A53 1987   616.85'5   87-22804

ISBN 1-879105-21-7

Printed in the United States of America

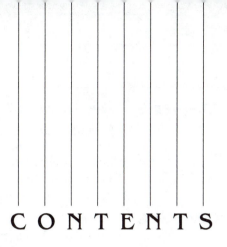

C O N T E N T S

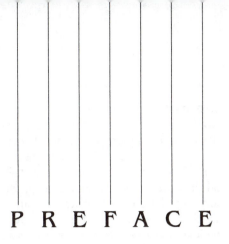

P R E F A C E

T he treatment of middle and high school students with voice disorders has been underemphasized by both training institutions and speech-language pathologists working in the field (Wilson, 1985). Some possible explanations for this neglect include (1) the lack of published material specific to this age group, (2) the assumption that the treatment of younger children is more productive (since problems are less habituated and therefore more responsive to intervention), and (3) the fact that few speech-language pathology programs require courses on normal adolescent development.

The passage of PL 94–142 (The Education for All Handicapped Children Act of 1975) mandated free and appropriate services to all handicapped students (including communicatively impaired) between the ages of 3 and 21. However, although speech-language pathologists now recognize their responsibility to service the adolescent population, many clinicians express a lack of confidence in working with this age group. Most have clinical experience primarily with younger children and/or with adults. Consequently, when faced with adolescents to treat, they often are forced to make adaptations of strategies previously used with different age groups.

Frequently, too, speech-language pathologists may be frustrated by what they perceive to be a lack of motivation on the part of the adolescent. Yet, it has been suggested that during puberty many students become motivated to make vocal changes because of increased needs of social acceptance (Wilson, 1985). A clinician's own knowledge, attitudes, and expectations concerning the efficacy of intervention with this population probably has a dramatic effect upon the outcome. To meet the needs of the adolescent population, speech-language pathologists need to have adequate information and resources available. Access to specific information relevant to the needs of these students enables speech-language pathologists to design and implement viable intervention programs.

Most voice disorders seen in adolescents (with the possible exception of mutational falsetto) are also seen in younger children and adults. Our central thesis is not that a specific disorder is unique to any population, but rather that an individual's needs, interests, and motivation are different at different stages of development. Thus, we believe that voice therapy programs should be designed *specifically* for adolescents. It is particularly important to recognize the interactive nature of adolescent development. Physical development occurs simultaneously with emotional and cognitive changes, all of which affect both each other and identity formation. Of course, the timing, sequence, and relative emphasis of the changes are unique to each individual.

Traditionally, textbooks of voice therapy have focused on descriptions and classifications of specific types of disorders and discussions of etiology. Therefore, this book will not concentrate on the readily accessible information of this kind. Rather, we will focus on the treatment of voice disorders specifically in adolescents. *Voice Therapy for Adolescents* was written particularly for practicing clinicians and clinicians in training. We assume that readers already have the general background and theoretical perspective necessary to explore the factors that influence program design for the adolescent population. Thus, we begin the book with a detailed discussion of the biological, psychosocial, and, of course, vocal changes that occur during adolescence. We then discuss various conditions that affect vocal behavior in adolescence, stressing interpersonal factors. Chapter 3 concentrates on the evaluation process in adolescents. In Chapter 4 we discuss contracting for treatment with adolescents, a particularly important aspect where motivation to change is concerned. Chapter 5 deals with the therapeutic process itself, especially in how the process is unique with the adolescent population. In Chapter 6 we bring the treatment process to a personal level, relating a number of case histories and interpreting their successes and failures based upon the interactive nature of treatment with adolescents.

The comprehensive Appendices to this book are, we feel, no less important than the text itself. The interested clinician will find here a large amount of practice materials for many diverse applications, as well as suggested activities for dealing with psychosocial problems that influence vocal problems. We have also included a bibliography of suggested readings relating to many topics relevant to working with the adolescent population.

Voice therapy for adolescents requires understanding of and sensitivity to many factors in addition to the vocal problems themselves. Speech-language clinicians have the capability of exerting a tremendous influence upon the emotional development of their clients, and such influence can, of course, be either positive or negative. *Voice Therapy for Adolescents* emphasizes above all the need for compassion and attention to the adolescent as a *person,* and stresses the enormous positive effect that the clinician can have upon an adolescent's development at this crucial time of life.

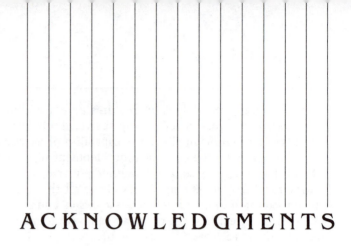

ACKNOWLEDGMENTS

We are indebted to many people for their encouragement and assistance. We are especially grateful to Marie Linvill and Susan Altman of College-Hill Press, and to Professor William H. Perkins, for their skilled direction in the preparation of this manuscript. We would also like to acknowledge our administrators, colleagues, and students at Indiana University and the Monroe County Community School Corporation, Bloomington, Indiana, for their support of this project.

We are especially appreciative of our parents, Roselyn Chamberlin and Noel and Verne Landsberg. They have provided an exemplary model of parenting at all stages of development.

Our husbands, Professors John O. Summers and R. Stansbury Stockton, in addition to being remarkably tolerant and understanding while we were working on this book, also provided astute academic insights. Finally, it is probably not coincidental that we undertook this project at a time when three very special young people, Alistair Andrews, Jill Summers, and Debra Summers, were in the process of teaching us so much, at close range, about adolescent behavior.

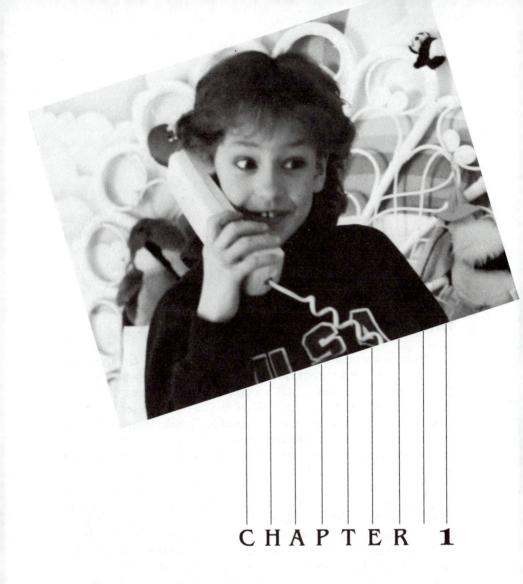

CHAPTER 1

Adolescence: A Time for Change

T he adolescent is neither a child nor an adult. Although some authorities refer to distinct stages during adolescent development and note the diverse needs of the age range, it is probably safe to generalize that all adolescents are in transition. They are experiencing dramatic changes in their bodies, in their social interactions, and in their lifestyles.

♦ PHYSICAL AND HORMONAL CHANGES

Most obvious in adolescence are the physical changes. They influence, to some extent, the emotional and sociological changes that occur as the individual redefines the self-concept. Changes include growth in height, growth of the sex organs leading to the capacity for reproduction, appearance of body hair, increased activity of sweat glands, increased secretion of skin oil, increased muscle mass and strength, and growth of the larynx, particularly an increase in the length of the vocal folds.

The predominant physical change that is of interest to voice clinicians working with adolescents is maturation of the laryngeal mechanism. Sometime during the middle/high school years boys and girls experience the hormonal changes that result in the physical manifestations of puberty. The time of onset and duration of puberty vary, but generally puberty occurs earlier in girls. However, vocal mutation, or the voice change that takes place as one manifestation of puberty, is more dramatic in boys than in girls. According to Aronson (1973), complete mutation of voice takes place within three to six months. During this time, the neck lengthens and the larynx increases in size and descends. The male vocal folds increase about 10 mm in length and become thicker. This increase in the size and mass of the folds influences the modal frequency of the voice, and a boy's pitch level lowers about an octave. Girls' vocal folds increase about 4 mm and their pitch levels lower about 3 to 4 semitones (Zemlin, 1968).

Most boys and girls go through voice change uneventfully. Generally, the changes in a girl's voice are not noticed. The majority of males also proceed through vocal mutation without the extreme vocal fluctuations and pitch breaks that society associates with the

2

stereotypical pubertal male. However, a boy may experience embarrassment when his increased laryngeal growth is not synchronized with neurological control of the changed structures and unpredictable vocal behaviors, such as unexpected pitch breaks, occur. However, to keep this in perspective, one study (Pedry, 1945) reported only four breaks in a total reading time of 84 hours for 1,014 adolescent boys. When Pedry questioned his subjects, 674 boys reported experiencing vocal breaks at some time and, of these, less than half remembered some feelings of embarrassment. Only six boys reported extreme embarrassment.

Derived from the Greek word *hormon*, meaning "to set in motion," hormones govern every aspect of growth and development as well as reproduction, metabolism, and emotional states. Hormones, which are secreted by the endocrine glands (thyroid, pituitary, adrenals, ovaries, and testes), interact in a complex manner that is still not completely understood. In adolescence, there is a sudden flooding of hormones into the bloodstream. The process starts with the master hormone, gonadotropin-releasing hormone (GRH), released in the hypothalamus. This signals the pituitary to secrete the gonadotropic hormones FSH (follicle-stimulating hormone) and LH (luteinizing hormone). These are called gonadotropic hormones because their targets are the gonads, or sex glands (ovaries in girls and testes in boys). FSH and LH cause the ovaries to produce estrogen and the testes to make testosterone. However, these sex hormones exert an additional influence on the brain, liver, salivary glands, skin, and muscles.

The human growth hormone (GH), produced by the pituitary, controls growth during childhood and puberty. The sexes appear to differ widely in the timing of the adolescent growth spurt, more so than in the age at which secondary sex characteristics appear. The growth spurt usually is the first overt sign of the onset of puberty, and longitudinal studies provide the most accurate information concerning the approximate range of ages at which each stage of puberty is reached. Boys develop, on the average, two years later than girls. The growth spurt occurs in American boys, on the average, at 14 years with the standard deviation of 0.9 years (Tanner, 1971). This peak velocity of height averages about 10.5 cm/year in boys. Children who have their peak early reach a height that is often somewhat higher than those who experience it late.

Changes in Boys

The adolescent growth spurt affects nearly all skeletal and muscular dimensions, but in different degrees. Leg length usually reaches its peak first, followed by body breadth and shoulder width. Increase in the muscle mass of the limbs and heart coincides with skeletal changes and with loss in fat. Boys also develop larger lungs relative to their overall size, which increases their respiratory capacity. Power, athletic skill, and physical endurance all increase rapidly throughout adolescence. Boys experience a greater increase in both muscle size and strength than girls, and this results in the ability to perform heavier tasks than girls can perform. Boys' physical endurance also increases.

Boys have greater increase in the length of their bones. Skeletal maturity, or "bone age," is frequently measured to ascertain developmental age. Skeletal maturity is closely related to the age at which adolescence (maturity measured by secondary sex characteristics) occurs. The physiological processes controlling skeletal development seem closely linked with those that initiate sexual maturation. Tempo of growth and maturation is biologically rooted but depends somewhat on an interaction of genetic and environmental factors (Tanner, 1971).

In boys, the earliest hormonal alterations of pubertal maturation involve secretion of the adrenal androgens — dehydroepilandrosterone and dehydroepiandrosterone sulfate. (Androgens are any substances that produce masculinizing effects. Others include androsterone and testosterone.) Plasma levels of these two hormones begin to rise between 6 and 10 years of age. Testosterone concentrations increase slightly by 11 years of age, while levels of pituitary gonadotropins, FSH and LH, increase slowly after age 8 to 10.

Although the timing of the onset of puberty varies, the sequence of events is usually strikingly similar between individuals. The first sign of puberty in boys is most often growth of the testes (Tanner, 1971). Male genital development, according to Marshall and Tanner (1970), is considered normal if it occurs between ages 9 and 15. However, male pubic hair growth in the absence of genital enlargement is sufficiently unusual to arouse suspicion of abnormality.

Growth of pubic hair (appearing about 18 months later in boys than in girls), height spurts, and penis growth usually begin approximately one year following the changes in the testes. The seminal vesicles and the prostate and bulbourethral glands develop and enlarge at the same time as penis growth occurs. About a year after penis development begins, there is the first ejaculation of seminal fluid.

Sebaceous and apocrine sweat glands develop rapidly in the skin of the male, and enlargement of the pores gives a coarser appearance to the skin, especially on the nose and limbs. Acne seems more common in boys than in girls because skin changes are related to androgenic activity. Male breast changes include an increase in the diameter of the areola and some temporary enlargement of breast tissue in some boys.

Axillary hair and facial hair do not generally appear until about two years after the onset of pubic hair growth. Although this is variable, there seems to be a definite pattern in the way the hairs of the mustache and beard occur. First, hair is seen at the corners, and then all over the upper lip. Next, hair is seen on the upper part of the cheeks, in the midline below the lower lip, and then along the sides and lower border of the chin. The amount of hair a boy finally acquires on his body seems to be related to heredity.

Since the appearance of facial hair in boys occurs toward the end of the sequence of physiological changes (e.g., genital development, height spurt, growth of pubic, axillary and facial hair), it is a useful reference point for the speech-language pathologist. Facial hair observed during a diagnostic session can indicate that the male student has reached the latter stages of pubertal maturation. Indeed, the speech-language pathologist who remembers the individual differences in boys' tempo of growth, yet is aware that the sequence of events remains consistent, would not be alarmed to note a high-pitched voice in a boy who obviously has not undergone a growth spurt or a low-pitched voice in a boy who obviously has. Between the ages of 9 and 14, the speech-language pathologist can expect greater variability as boys begin the sequence of pubertal changes. The diagnostician must have the flexibility to observe indications of skeletal and maturational levels.

Enlargement of the larynx and lengthening of the vocal folds usually occur relatively late in the maturational process (e.g., after the onset of genital changes). This is caused by the action of testosterone on the laryngeal cartilages (Tanner, 1971) and affects pitch level and variability. Quality changes in the male voice are related to increased respiratory capacity and enlargement of the resonating cavities above the larynx. The increased resonance capacity is related to adolescent enlargement of the nose, mouth, and maxilla. The observant speech-language pathologist may detect, for example, "adolescent facies" that are associated with the structural growth of the oronasal areas.

Changes in Girls

Girls complete the adolescent growth spurt earlier than boys (at about age 11 to 13 for girls, versus as late as about 15 for boys). The peak velocity of height (PHV, which is used extensively in growth studies) averages about 9 cm/year (Tanner, 1971). The velocity over the whole year encompassing the six months before and after the peak is somewhat less. During this year, girls usually grow between 6 and 11 cm (in contrast to boys who grow between 7 and 12 cm). Nearly all skeletal and muscular dimensions are involved in the dramatic growth spurt, though not, of course, to the same degree. The earliest structures to reach their adult size are the head, hands, and feet. Many adolescent girls complain about having big hands and feet, and many parents note that in fights with siblings, adolescents do not always realize their hand strength. Leg length usually reaches its peak next, followed by body breadth and shoulder width. Most of the spurt in height is due to acceleration of trunk length rather than leg length. The increase in muscle mass coincides with skeletal growth. Girls, because they experience their spurt earlier, may have a period when their muscles are larger than those of their male contemporaries. However, once the growth spurt has occurred in males, they become stronger than females. They have larger muscles, hearts, and lungs and a higher systolic blood pressure. Boys lose fat during the growth spurt, whereas it merely decelerates in girls.

Although the sebaceous and apocrine sweat glands develop rapidly during puberty, this is usually less marked in girls than in boys. In girls, the appearance of the "breast bud" is usually the first sign of puberty, though the appearance of pubic hair may precede it in about one-third of the adolescent female population. Both the uterus and vagina develop at the same time as the breast, and the labia and clitoris also enlarge. These developments precede menarche (the first menstruation), which occurs relatively late in the maturation sequence, and rarely begins before the height spurt has been achieved. On the average, girls grow only about 6 cm more after menarche (Tanner, 1971). During the adolescent growth spurt, a girl's body composition shows a ratio of lean to fat tissue of 5:1. At menarche, this ratio has reached 3:1. At the average age of menarche (between the 12th and 13th birthdays) 24 percent of a girl's body composition is fat, and her critical weight is between 94 and 103 pounds (Frisch and Revelle, 1971). Naturally there is tremendous normal variation that occurs in the interval from the appearance of the first sign of puberty to complete maturity (from 18 months to 6 years). Marshall and Tanner (1969) provide an excellent summary of the limits of what may be considered normal.

The sequence of biological changes that occurs at adolescence has not changed over centuries. However, the time of onset has changed markedly. Improved social conditions and improved nutrition across socioeconomic levels have resulted in less variation in onset as a function of class status. Much of the variation that still exists could probably be attributed to genetic factors. However, it has frequently been observed that girls in warmer climates (e.g., Mediterranean cultures) mature earlier than those in less temperate climates. Modern writers relate these differences to dietary practices rather than to geographic influences such as temperature and light exposure.

Since the publication of Frisch's (1971) studies on critical weights, attention has been focused on the role of exercise on the biological development of the female adolescent. Legislation (e.g., Title IX) that mandated equal opportunity for female high school students has, in many instances, improved the physical education programs available for girls. In view of the earlier age of onset of menarche in present day society and concerns about high pregnancy rates among teenagers, many experts feel that sedentary lifestyles, in combination with rich diets, could be responsible for the shift toward fertility at earlier ages. To combat this trend, some educators are committed to providing courses in nutrition and regular exercise for all female students in the middle and high schools. However, when female athletes and dancers exercise to the point where critical body ratios are jeopardized, cessation of menstrual periods can occur.

The most widespread concern of middle and high school girls is learning to deal with the discomfort associated with managing their early menstrual cycles while maintaining active teenage lifestyles. Some girls experience severe menstrual pain, cramping, and irregular, unpredictable cycles. Increased anxiety, irritability, and mood swings can occur in the week or so preceding the onset of the menstrual flow. A cluster of symptoms associated with this time in the female cycle has been categorized as premenstrual syndrome (Dalton, 1977).

It is documented that as many as 95 percent of women experience some symptoms of premenstrual syndrome, or PMS (e.g., depression, fatigue, irritability, anxiety, edema of laryngeal and nasal mucosa, acne, breast soreness, or bloating) in the week or so preceding their menstrual flow. The intensity of discomfort during the menstrual cycle may be influenced by the circumstances in which it is experienced. Some physicians have postulated that PMS is due to the tension of modern life, but studies of cultures throughout the world dispute this hyposthesis, and definitive evidence concerning the exact cause of PMS still eludes researchers.

Occasionally, the speech-language pathologist may encounter female students with cyclical vocal symptoms that may be related to the menstrual cycle — lowered pitch, hoarseness, vocal instability, voice "breaks," huskiness, sinus/nasal congestion, and decreased flexibility in the upper part of the singing range. It is possible also that some individuals may be especially sensitive to the effects of synthetic hormones (such as those in birth control pills) on the phonatory system. Many professional voice users avoid use of contraceptive pills, which are made up of synthetic estrogen and progestin, because they believe the changes that occur in the vocal mechanism seriously affect vocal quality and artistic performance. It is also interesting to note that it has long been the custom in European opera houses for female singers to have the option of not performing during those times in the menstrual cycle when their voices are adversely affected. Usually, however, the effects of the menstrual cycle on the voice are subtle and may not be significant unless the young woman has a great investment in activities involving aesthetic vocal performance.

There is some evidence that premenstrual swelling of the laryngeal and nasal membranes contributes to voice quality deviations. Women who experience severe vocal problems will require a comprehensive medical evaluation by a physician who is knowledgeable concerning PMS. They may also need assistance in monitoring fluctuations in specific symptoms. Lifestyle changes (e.g., stress reduction techniques, dietary modifications to reduce fluid retention in tissues, and exercise) are frequently suggested as management strategies. Each individual needs to monitor her own reactions and learn optimum ways of managing symptoms. For example, avoiding vocally abusive activities when laryngeal edema is present may be especially important for students who aspire to professional voice use.

♦ HORMONAL THERAPY

Reiter (1981) reported that delayed adolescence occurs in 25 of every thousand children; in 2 to 5 percent of males, sexual development will be delayed more than 2 years, and in 0 to 1 percent more than 3 years. However, unless the physical growth spurt has occurred, physicians frequently may not think about delayed sexual maturation.

If the adult stage of genital development has not occurred by the age of 17, physicians usually consider the possibility of systemic or endocrinologic disease. However, there can be a familial pattern of constitutional delay where the timing of pubertal events is shifted to a later time. Sometimes this may be related to nutritional deprivation or psychological aberrations within the family.

Physicians use hormonal therapy to treat adolescents with delayed or disturbed growth and sexual development. There seems to be some evidence that stress hormones can suppress growth and may be linked to depression, upper respiratory infections, cancers, and memory loss. Some researchers believe that teenagers who mature late and have adjustment problems may have higher levels of cortisol (an adrenal cortical hormone).

Close medical supervision is required in all instances of hormonal therapy because of the vast array of side effects that can occur. Currently, the major reasons for hormone usage in the adolescent age group include treatment of medical conditions, birth control, and improved athletic performance.

Testosterone, a male hormone, is classified as a steroid (which resembles cholesterol compounds) rather than as a protein hormone. The functions of testosterone are (1) the androgenic, or masculinizing effect, (2) the anabolic, or protein-building effect, and (3) an inhibitory effect on the hypophysis (pituitary gland) (Witzmann, 1977). When the body does not produce enough male hormone, such as in children with chromosomal abnormalities, testosterone replacement therapy is frequently the only means of clincal intervention designed to stimulate sexual development and the emergence of the male secondary sex characteristics. In cases such as kidney disorders and slow-healing fractures, the protein-building effect may be used therapeutically. However, with these patients, the body is already producing testosterone at the appropriate level for the individual. Therefore, the added steroid hormone almost always produces some adverse effects directly proportional to the dosage and length of treatment. Occasionally, testosterone is administered clinically in order to produce an inhibitory effect upon hormone production. This occurs because the hypophysis is part of the body's mechanism for regulating hormone production and, in the presence of increased hormones, the hypophysis will send the message for the body to reduce production of that hormone.

It is impossible to completely separate the three functions of testosterone. Almost all testosterone recipients experience the hormone's androgenic, anabolic, and inhibitory effects, as well as the substance's adverse side effects. There is general agreement that prolonged ingestion of very large doses of testosterone does increase lean body mass and total body weight. Thus, for the athlete, this may appear to be an easy way to increase overall athletic strength. However, when a male ingests large doses of synthetic testosterone, the testes stop producing their own testosterone. Paradoxically, even though a large amount of synthetic testosterone is present in the blood, a cessation of natural testosterone results in a feminizing effect.

If high doses of testosterone are given to a prepubescent male, (e.g., a junior high football player who is under pressure to gain weight and muscle mass quickly), the results may be disastrous. The physical changes (appearance of facial and pubic hair, increase in height, increase in vocal fold size resulting in a deepening of the voice, and the production of testosterone) may occur only partially, if at all. This is because the hypothalamus monitors the level of testosterone in the body rather than specific physical changes. Thus, in the presence of high levels of exogenous testosterone, the hypothalamus sends messages to the target organs saying, "OK, puberty is over. You can stop growing facial and pubic hair, close the growth plates, and stop lengthening the vocal folds." The boy may be only 12 years old and 5 feet tall and not yet through puberty, but the hypothalamus has done its job. As a result, the boy will probably grow up to be several inches shorter than he would have been if he had not taken testosterone. He may not develop facial and pubic hair, and he will probably go through voice change (vocal mutation) at a late age, if at all.

Androgenic (masculinizing and virilizing) effects of testosterone on females may include menstrual disturbances, coarsening of the skin, male hair-growth patterns or baldness, and a deepening of the voice.

Some of the signs of steroid use include impatience, hostility, increased sex drive, less sleep, aging skin, head hair loss, increased body hair, darker colored genitals, and collection of cholesterol globules on the underside of the eyeballs (Todd, 1983; Jerome, 1980). Possible side effects from steroid use include sterility, liver problems, and atherosclerosis (Todd, 1983).

Jerome (1980) stated that birth control pills are, in themselves, steroids. Oral contraceptives contain synthetic forms of estrogen and progesterone. These externally supplied hormones assume some of the functions of the internally produced hormones, but block others. For example, the synthetic estrogen and progesterone in oral contraceptives build up the uterine lining, but suppress ovulation. They have been used not only to control fertility, but also to ameliorate menstrual pain.

◆ **VOCAL MUTATION**

Aristotle was probably the first writer who definitely connected voice change with puberty. Prepubertal male and female larynges are the same size. At puberty, the larynx descends and the dimensions of the infraglottal sagittal and transverse planes increase. The anterioposterior dimensions also increase, with greater increases in the male larynx than in the female larynx. The angle of the male thyroid lamina decreases to 90 degrees compared with the female angle of 120 degrees (Aronson, 1980). The vocal folds increase in length, the mucosa becomes stronger, and the epiglottis increases in size.

Kahane (1978) reported measurements he made from 10 white male and 10 white female cadaveric larynges, ranging in age from 9 to 18 years at death. He compared his findings with the relatively few other studies of the human circumpubertal larynx reported in the literature. When Kahane compared his prepubertal and pubertal groups, he consistently observed several morphological relationships:

♦ Pubertal cartilage and soft tissue measurements were significantly larger than prepubertal measurements for both sexes, although within-sex differences were greater among males than among females.

♦ Sex differences were not present before puberty (first noted by Klock, 1968). Some of the differences noted included:
   1. Length of vocal folds and weights of laryngeal cartilages were significantly larger in pubertal males than in pubertal females.
   2. Thyroid eminence in pubertal males was more prominent than in pubertal females.
   Kahane believed that his measurements of the cricoid, arytenoid, and soft tissues also supported the notion that there is significantly greater growth in the larynx of the male than in the larynx of the female from prepuberty to puberty.

♦ Pubertal laryngeal measurements in both sexes, however, were still clearly different from adults in seven dimensions:
   1. The weights of all laryngeal cartilages.
   2. The angle of the thyroid laminae (regional growth in the male thyroid cartilage appeared to take place in the anterior aspect).
   3. The height of the cricoid arch, anteriorly at midline.
   4. Distance between the cricoid facets.
   5. Midsagittal length of the cricoid lumen.
   6. Superolateral length of the cricoid.
   7. Anterior ridge height of the arytenoid cartilages.

Since the prepubertal female dimensions more clearly approximate adult size and weight, Kahane (1978) extrapolated that the prepubertal female requires less laryngeal growth per unit of time to mature than does the prepubertal male. Sizable differences found in the weights of adult and pubertal cartilages led to the conclusion that differences were probably related to ossification that may begin as early as 20 years of age (Hately, Evison, & Samuel, 1965). In contrast, the length of both male and female vocal folds at puberty was not significantly different from that of adults (measurements of vocal fold length were "total or inclusive," not merely the membranous portion). The amount of increase in vocal fold length in the male was 10.87 mm and 4.16 mm in the female. Kahane noted that the greater growth in the length of the male folds is probably accompanied by increases in width, although this dimension was not explored in this study. The greater structural changes in the male larynx correlate with the greater drop in fundamental frequency of the male voice during puberty.

Weiss (1950) in his classic study, listed several changes within the organs of phonation during pubertal development of the male:

♦ The lungs undergo a large increase in breathing capacity. Both the circumference and length of the chest cavity increase rapidly.

♦ The neck increases in length and width. When the neck lengthens, the larynx descends relative to this growth. This increases the length and width of the pharyngeal tube. Weiss claimed a widening of the oral pharynx during this time, coupled with the change of length in the pharyngeal cavity, causes the change of vocal timbre.

♦ There is relatively little material available in regard to the pubertal development of the nasal sinuses. Some sinuses do not appear until this time, especially the frontal sinuses. The addition of these sinuses gives more resonance and a distinct quality to the voice.

♦ The larynx enlarges considerably due to the influence of sex hormones. The concept that the larynx increases to double its size is false. This idea was derived from the belief that the pitch of the voice depends upon the length of the vocal cords, and since male voices generally descend one octave, the cords must double in size. The length of the vocal lips within the larynx grow by about 1 cm in males and about 3 to 4 mm in females.

Weiss (1950) determined that the main difference between pubertal development in males and females concerned the main direction of the growth of the larynx. Until puberty, they are essentially the same size, but during pubertal growth, the male larynx grows especially fast in the anterioposterior direction. This results in the "protrusion of what is known as the 'pommmum Adami' (Adam's Apple), the distinct lengthening of the vocal cords and the narrowing of the angle formed by both plates of the thyroid cartilage. All these features are more pronounced in individuals with deep voices, and may appear even in females in that same category" (p. 131). Generally, the female larynx grows more in height than in width or depth at this stage and becomes distinctly different from the male larynx.

Weiss (1950) claimed an overall increase in the size of all organs of phonation. This results in a deepening of the voice and an increase in breath and resonance with more vocal power. The range of descent averages an octave for males and 3 to 4 notes for females. Weiss mentioned further physical transformation that takes place during this mutation: "The mucosa of the larynx becomes stronger and less transparent. The tonsils and adenoids atrophy (decrease in size) to a certain degree. The cavernous tissue of the nasal turbinates develops. The epiglottis increases in size, flattens out, and assumes a more elevated position" (p. 132).

Weiss (1950) felt that there were certain "premutational" changes, including some loss of voice, a slight lowering of pitch, and problems controlling the voice. The "huskiness" has been noted by many writers and may be due to incomplete closure of the glottis (posterior glottal chink) before the folds complete the thickening and lengthening process. It is generally believed that the speaking voice completes mutation within about three to six months, but that the singing voice may take one to two years to completely mature.

Tosi, Postan, and Bianculli (1976) studied male children in Buenos Aires over an eight-month period. They found that at mean age 13.3 years, their subjects showed maximal change of fundamental frequency and minimal value of standard deviation (17 Hz).

A study of pitch changes by McGlone and Hollien (1963) demonstrated that female voices lowered 2.4 semitones during puberty. At completion of vocal mutation, the female average fundamental frequencies found by Mischel et al. (1966) were 277 Hz. Hollien and Malcik (1967) reported the median fundamental frequency of 18-year-old males was 126 Hz. In an earlier study by Curry (1940), 10-year-old boys had a median fundamental frequency of 269 Hz, and 14-year-old boys had a median of 241 Hz, with 18-year-olds dropping to 137 Hz. Hollien and Malcik (1967) and Hollien, Malcik, and Hollien (1965) studied southern males and reported lower median fundamental frequency levels for adolescent black males.

Andrews (1982) tested 740 Australian school children aged 5 to 13 years and analyzed vocal frequency measurements in relation to age, sex, weight, height, and neck circumference. A significant difference between boys' and girls' measurements appeared at age 9.5 years. When the children were divided into two groups (i.e., 5 to 9.5 years old and 9.5 to 13 years old), an analysis of variance indicated that with respect to habitual levels of the younger group, height, weight, neck circumference, sex, and age (and the interaction between sex and age) were not significant. However, weight was significant ($F = 6.030$, $p < .015$). For the older group, sex was highly significant ($F = 23.280$, $p < .001$) as was height ($F = 4.548, p < .034$). These results underscore the relationship between habitual frequency level, sex, and height as the child matures. As children grow older, height may be a more useful index of vocal maturity than chronological age. Neck circumference did not correlate with frequency measurements in this study.

Two methods of eliciting measurements of basal frequency were compared in Andrews' (1982) study. One method involved sliding down to the lowest possible pitch (visual feedback was provided on the Visi-Pitch screen), and the other method was the traditional approach of asking children to produce their lowest pitch (visual feedback was also provided). Three trials were given for each approach. It is interesting to note that for all age groups, the sliding method of obtaining basal frequency resulted in measurements that averaged 20 Hz lower than those obtained using the traditional method of elicitation. For example, the 12- to 13-year-old children produced an average basal frequency of 208 Hz when asked to produce their lowest note, yet "slid down" to an average basal pitch of 187 Hz. It seemed as if it was easier for these students to "descend" to their basal pitch than to "land" on it. One is reminded of how untrained singers sometimes seem to "slide down" to the lower notes in their range.

When basal frequency measurements were compared with habitual frequency levels for all children in the study, there was an average of 43 Hz difference between the two measures, whereas the lowest limit of the conversational pitch range they used averaged 23 Hz below the habitual average level. A summary of the habitual and basal levels of the students aged 9 to 13 years appears in Table 1–1. It may be that basal pitch measures reflect laryngeal change earlier than do habitual pitch measures, since lower notes may be added to the available range prior to the adoption of a lower habitual level.

A technique that is sometimes helpful in facilitating production of basal pitch is to ask students to "slide down" into vocal fry, the lowest frequency register characterized by a rough vocal quality. Some high school choir directors may at times even encourage male students to sing low notes with fry. The technique is referred to as the "Russian" method, since Russian bass voices are noted for depth and richness of tone. Teachers of singing also use the term *low terminal pitch* when referring to the basal or lowest musical note in an individual's range of available pitches.

During the 19th century in Italy, castration was frequently practiced to maintain the childlike soprano voice in male singers. The castrati had pure high-pitched voices due to their immature laryngeal

TABLE 1-1.

Averaged Measurements of Habitual and Basal Frequency Levels During Early Adolescence

Age	No.	Habitual Level (Hz)	Basal Level (Hz)
Boys			
9 years	68	237	192
10 years	67	226	191
11 years	92	227	186
12 years	30	225	182
13 years	32	221	180
Girls			
9 years	55	236	199
10 years	49	237	196
11 years	70	237	196
12 years	26	236	192
13 years	31	227	191

development, combined with the respiratory capacity of an adult male. Nowadays, rather than attempting to prevent voice change in male singers, choir directors and teachers of singing work to ensure a careful transition from the child's singing voice to mature male voice. There has been a great deal of controversy concerning whether adolescent males should sing during their period of voice change, and the type of singing that should be encouraged. Writers such as Cooper (1970), Swanson (1960), and McKenzie (1956) have presented differing views concerning the way the singing voices of adolescent males should be treated. Whereas the speaking voice has a mutational duration of three to six months, the singing voice can take longer, perhaps up to two years. This vocal mutation generally follows a predictable pattern during puberty: from soprano to alto (11 to 12 years of age), to a cross between alto and baritone (13 to 14 years of age), to light baritone (14 to 15 years of age), and, finally, to a more settled baritone, bass, or tenor (16 to 19 years of age).

Joseph (1963) studied 200 adolescent males (aged 11 years 10 months to 16 years 9 months) and tape recorded them once monthly for eight consecutive months. The average low terminal pitch at the start of the study was around C to C# on the bass staff. This average lowered to a low A on the bass staff, or by about a third, during the 8-month test. The average boy's range at the beginning of the study was 1⅓ octaves, while the median range was 1⅕ octaves. The average range at the end of the study was 2⅓ octaves, while the median range was 2 octaves and 1 second.

Naidr, Zobril and Sevcik (1965) in Czechoslovakia performed a longitudinal study of male adolescent voice mutation. On the average, the most significant changes took place during ages 13 and 14. The lower limit of the singing range lowered eight semitones, and the upper limit lowered 13 semitones. Cooksey (1977) provides a detailed summary of changes in the singing voice of the adolescent male.

♦ **PSYCHOSOCIAL FACTORS RELATED TO PHYSICAL MATURATION**

Teenagers are in the process of acquiring new body images. Pubescent males and females are busy "trying out" new social roles and their attention, quite naturally, is focused on comparisons of their own bodies with those of others. Their degree of physical maturation affects the perceptions adults, as well as peers, have of them, so environmental reinforcers interact with somatic changes. Money and Clopper (1974) break down "psychosocial" age into academic, recreational, and psychosexual age. These usually correlate with chronological and physique age. When deviations from the usual timetable of pubertal development occur, the predictable psychosocial adjustments of adolescence are more difficult.

Physical changes and the wide variability that exists among individuals when these changes occur affect the adolescent's body image, which is closely related to self-esteem. It is important to note that body image is not objective. It is affected by how the individual perceives others' reactions and by society's concept of the "ideal body." Adolescent anxiety is generated by real or imagined defects and differences in physical characteristics. A number of studies have reported how males and females are affected differently by early or late maturation (Grinder, 1973; Hamachek, 1973; McCandless & Coop, 1979; Miller, 1974; Mussen & Jones, 1957, Tanner, 1971). Boys who approach adult height and muscle power early seem to be more successful in sports (Espenschade & Eckert, 1967). They are more likely to be accepted and treated by peers and adults as more psychologically and socially mature. Early-maturing boys are more often chosen as leaders and as dates (Jones, 1958). However, adults may thrust responsibility onto a boy whose physical appearance is mature and expect mature social and emotional responses before those facets of the child's development are complete. Although adolescents who mature early are likely to be given opportunities to learn responsibility, late-maturing adolescents may be given fewer opportunities to demonstrate mature behaviors. The late-maturing male may feel insecure and inferior and may be perceived as more dependent and rebellious (Mussen & Jones, 1957). Early maturers may seem more independent and mature in interpersonal relations. There is some evidence to suggest that these personality and behavioral differences may persist into adulthood (Grinder, 1973; Jones, 1965).

Differences between early- and late-maturing girls, although similar to those noted in boys, seem neither as dramatic nor as long lasting (Hamacheck, 1973; Jones & Mussen, 1958). An early-maturing girl may be disadvantaged, initially, if her peer group is less mature and her parents treat her as a "little girl" (Kiell, 1964). However, as her peers catch up with her, this disadvantage disappears, and she may, in fact, be admired by them. A late-maturing girl may develop problems with interpersonal relations and may develop a negative self-concept, but, again, these disadvantages dissipate as she, too, matures and shares experiences and interests. Girls are sometimes perceived to be less stigmatized by deviant rates of development than are boys in our culture since the female sex role has been less clearly defined (Hamachek, 1973; McCandless & Coop, 1979). Although girls are judged more frequently on their appearance, they also have the advantage of being able to modify appearance with the help of cosmetics and foundation garments.

Dobson (1978) stated that feelings of inferiority plague the majority of adolescents. He believed that there are three things that cause great anxiety and depression for teenagers: physical attractiveness, intelligence, and money. Most teenagers also have difficulties with the jumble of emotions they sometimes experience at the same moment. For example, they may have difficulties with special occasions when expectations collide with disappointments or fears.

Teenagers face a wide array of adult experiences and problems for the first time, and many of them have trouble dealing with mistakes. It is hard to hold on to self-esteem in the face of what seems like miserable failure. Their reaction to accumulated frustrations is frequently a feeling of powerlessness. Problems and decisions take on major proportions not always commensurate with reality. To assuage the frightening feelings of inadequacy that engulf them at such times, teenagers need a tremendous amount of encouragement and understanding from adults to "shore up" their shaky self-images. It's imperative that they have helpful, supportive adults to talk to and learn from. This enables them to hear some "good things" about themselves and to build self-confidence.

One of the major tasks of adolescence is to learn to experience intense feelings and to express them appropriately. Adolescents need adult models, structure, and opportunities for trial and error as they develop coping strategies. They need reassurance that in their confusion and moodiness, they are not alone.

Depression

A healthy adolescence is characterized by variability in emotional state, and balance between activity and privacy. Although the vast majority of adolescents develop methods for coping with stress through trial and error, some, unfortunately, do not. Serious depression affects 1 person in 5 at some time (Zehr, 1983). This is not the same as ordinary unhappiness, but a persistent mood that affects a person's basic emotional disposition.

Acute or "reactive" depression is precipitated by an event that occurs in the normal course of life. A loss of a loved one or loss of possessions or opportunities are predictable triggers of acute depression. Adolescents who "break up" with friends, fail exams, or don't make the team experience forms of acute depression, which is intense and painful, but short lived. It is frequently a strengthening experience that leaves the individual with greater insight and flexibility. Usually within 6 months to 1 year after the event, an individual is able to place it in perspective. The loss may still be felt, but its effect is no longer debilitating.

Chronic depression is harder to explain than depression related to a specific event or loss, and often seems associated with a person's mood or temperament. A chronically depressed person may deny the effects of a traumatic event and block out the experience. It is common in chronic depression for there to be a delay between an event responsible for it and the first signs of mood change. Young women who have been raped or sexually harassed sometimes appear to handle the aftermath "calmly" and are proud of their ability to do so. Later, other difficulties (such as examinations or financial problems) may appear to create major depression, and help may then be sought for a problem that postdates the real cause of the depression.

Chronic depression may be related to family problems, such as divorce or alcoholism, where the adolescent feels responsibility for another person's pain and self-destructiveness. Children of alcoholics or of other substance abusers frequently exhibit coping strategies that are related to their dysfunctional family lives (Wegscheider-Cruse, 1983). Because in our culture families afflicted with alcoholism tend to conceal or deny it, adolescent children of alcoholic parents frequently do not receive the assistance they need. This occurs at a time in the adolescent's life when support and emotional stability at home are vital to emotional growth and development.

Divorce, the adjustments required in families combined by new marriages, violence in the home, and rape (especially date-rape in this age group) all constitute major emotional traumas that threaten the very core of the adolescent's self-esteem. All will engender some degree of loss and grief. Loss and grief are complex processes involving many emotions and coping strategies. The adolescent personality, which is already unstable, is particularly vulnerable to the effect of loss. Loss of security may be felt by an adolescent who moves to a new school or community or who loses some function or ability through accident or illness. Any aspect of the lifestyle that is curtailed can be the impetus for depression. Loss of sources of satisfaction and stability threaten a student's overall feelings of security and worth. Individuals deal with loss and grief in different ways; however, Kubler-Ross (1969) listed five stages that she believed were consistently seen: denial, anger, bargaining, depression, and acceptance.

An adolescent's inability to cope with normal developmental stresses (sex-role definition, emerging independence, the inability to tolerate temporary frustration in order to gain long-term satisfaction) may result in serious depression. The statistics on teenage suicide in the United States indicate that this is a problem that cannot be ignored.

The suicide rate for young people has tripled in the last 10 years, and suicide is usually a cry for help (Bell, 1980). Eight out of ten people who commit suicide tell someone that they're thinking about suicide before they actually attempt it. When a student talks about suicide, it is important not to change the subject. A person who mentions suicide should be taken seriously and given a chance to express his or her feelings. Warning signs of severe depression include:

♦ A noticeable change in eating and sleeping habits.
♦ A loss of interest in friends.
♦ Feelings of hopelessness and self-hate.
♦ Constant restlessness and hyperactivity.
♦ Significant change in school performance.
♦ Verbalization of a plan for suicide.
♦ Possession of a weapon or pills.
♦ Giving away of prized possessions.
♦ A long and deep reaction to a breakup or death.

Fantasies of revenge are frequent among teenagers with suicidal thoughts. Counselors who encourage teenagers to verbalize their thoughts of loss and revenge use techniques such as "Imagine your own funeral" and "Imagine how bad they'll feel after you're gone." Bell (1980) noted that feelings about people's reactions to a fantasized suicide can generate ideas about how the adolescent would like things to be different. Fantasies of loss and revenge are frequently mixed with strong feelings about being alive. Communicating these feelings can help troubled adolescents develop techniques for changing or escaping suicidal thoughts.

Cognitive and Psychosocial Factors

Adolescents are ideal candidates for voice therapy because they have the cognitive development to deal with the ideas and concepts related to modification of behavior. Adolescents have the ability to think abstractly, to develop hypothetical solutions to problems, and to test solutions against the evidence. They are able to consider not only what is, but what might be. The behavior and beliefs of adolescents are influenced by many factors, including the socioeconomic status of their families, the quality of schooling, individual personality characteristics, psychosocial factors, and emerging independence from parents. Naturally, there are some adolescents who do not achieve the more advanced levels of cognitive functioning because of intellectual, cultural, or experiential constraints. Cognitive development significantly influences how adolescents think about themselves, their families, peers, and society.

Emerging cognitive abilities may cause friction between adolescents and significant adults. Once an adolescent has the cognitive ability to consider things "as they might be," impatience and criticism of reality result. Parents, school, therapy, home life, and societal values frequently are the targets of criticism when they differ from what the adolescent considers to be the ideal.

Many adolescents with well-developed cognitive skills are idealists critical of the existing social order. They propose solutions that may be unrealistic, and question authority without always having the responsibility for implementing their ideas. The capability to examine a number of ideas simultaneously and to point out inconsistencies is characteristic of the adolescent's maturing cognitive abilities. Since adolescents can conceive of and consider many alternative solutions to a problem, they are capable of perceiving a variety of options to behavioral and interpersonal skills. Generating a variety of options enhances student participation in the voice therapy process.

Defense Mechanisms

Defense mechanisms are unconscious means for dealing with anxiety (Laughlin, 1970). Two defense mechanisms which first appear in adolescence are intellectualization and asceticism (Conger, 1973; Muuss, 1975; Bloss, 1962). Intellectualization involves dealing with emotional matters on an intellectual plane so that instinctual drives can be consciously controlled. Asceticism is an attempt to deny instinctual drives, such as sex and hunger, and it sometimes provides group support for self-denial. Some writers consider asceticism to be a negative strategy because it prevents adolescents from coming to terms with their instinctual drives. Intellectualization, when carried to excess, may result in social isolation and may serve as a way to avoid coping directly with needs and conflicts. On the other hand, intellectualizing problems provides useful experience in hypothetical and abstract thinking. It may also help an adolescent deal with instinctual drives realistically.

Egocentrism

Elkind (1967) believed that since an adolescent's thoughts are mainly self-centered, he or she therefore assumes that other people are equally obsessed with his or her behavior and appearance. Adolescents feel they are the focus of everyone's attention, which increases feelings of self-consciousness. This may result at times in a fear of exposure to the criticism of others, which leads to an increased desire for privacy. Elkind also believed that an adolescent's egocentric cognitive processes may lead to over-differentiation concerning feelings. The adolescent may believe that no one else has felt such important or special agony or rapture. Adolescent egocentrism is broken down as the young person observes, listens, and talks to others and discovers that peers share similar feelings and concerns. However, some adolescents' sense of uniqueness extends beyond the feeling domain to other areas and may result in dangerous activities. For example, if a girl feels that her feelings, her person and, indeed, her fate are unique to the extent that accidents, rape, pregnancy and death happen only to others, the consequences may be very unfortunate. Some adolescents, however, assume instead that the world is indifferent. Consequently, bids for attention may be made to shore up feelings of inadequacy. Kagan (1971) believed that adolescents are anxious about living up to, and not violating, the standards of society.

Moral Development

Kohlberg (1975) stated that there are three levels of morality: the preconventional, the conventional, and the postconventional. He expanded on Piaget's work (1974) and related moral development to Piaget's cognitive theory.

The preconventional level of morality corresponds to Piaget's stage of concrete thought and is generally seen in middle-class children from 4 to 10 years of age. At this stage goodness and badness are considered in terms of physical consequences and the physical power of authority figures. The child behaves because of fear of punishment and desire for reward. Conventional morality initially appears and then dominates moral judgment during preadolescence; morality is equated with social approval and the maintenance of law and order to avoid guilt and penalties. The postconventional level does not appear until adolescence and corresponds to a higher level in Piaget's stage of formal thought. Here, morality does not rely on obedience, conformity, and social approval, but rather on universal principles of justice. However, it is probably true that the need for peer acceptance, as well as increased sexual and aggressive urges, often influence the decision-making more strongly than do moral values. At age 12 or 13, a young person usually moves from a protected elementary school environment to a middle or junior high school, where an increasing number of moral dilemmas are encountered.

The Role of Peers

In Western cultures, the peer group is an important factor in the maturation process during adolescence. Peers help support a young person's growing autonomy by allowing experimentation with new roles and providing reassurance and psychological security.

Peer groups tend to be chosen because of similarities, rather than differences, and help define identity. Adolescents receive more comfort from peers who are simultaneously experiencing the same anxieties and concerns, and, in this sense, the peer group can be therapeutic (Conger, 1973). The intimacy of the peer group allows the expression of hostile, guilty, and resentful feelings associated with school, sexuality, disobedience, parental restrictions, and the ambiguous future that cannot be shared with significant adults (Osterrieth, 1969). Comfort from peers, although important for all adolescents, is especially critical for those who have inadequate support in the family environment. Although concerned, supportive parents are primary sources of high self-esteem, acceptance and admiration by peers provide objective sources for feelings of self-worth. Peer evaluation may be especially important in the young person's self-perception, since the roles played at this vulnerable stage of development may have long-term ramifications. Material benefits, such as a car, money, or clothes, may contribute to an individual's sense of power within the group. In addition, personality characteristics and physical and mental skill have an effect on perceived power within groups.

The peer group allows the adolescent to learn more mature ways of relating to both sexes (Winder, 1974). Sex role identity, though learned in the context of the family, is reinforced within the context of the peer group (Mischel, 1970). Intense friendships develop during adolescence. During childhood, the choice of friends is influenced most by proximity and the focus is on activity, whereas during adolescence, the focus is on interpersonal involvement (Douvan & Adelson, 1966). Although both boys and girls have intimate friendships, these relationships are more intense among girls, since boys are usually socialized toward achievement, action, and the attainment of power.

Since the adolescent's values tend to be learned within the family, the peer group chosen will often reflect the socioeconomic class, values, and morality of the family.

Styles of Parenting

It is important for the speech-language pathologist to understand parenting styles for three reasons: (1) The dynamics existing within an adolescent's family frequently affect the student's reactions to other adults. (2) Teachers and counselors frequently adopt recognizable parenting styles during interactions with students. (3) Frequently it is necessary for the speech-language pathologist to monitor his or her style and adapt it to the needs of individual students.

Parenting styles may exist on a continuum. At one extreme is the authoritarian parent, and at the other is the permissive parent. Authoritarian parenting thwarts self-mastery and decision-making ability, encouraging conformity to external demands. Permissive parents, on the other hand, carry acceptance to an extreme, making very few demands of any sort on the child. This attitude may hinder development of self-esteem and decision-making ability. At the midpoint in the continuum is the "authoritative" parent. Many researchers believe the authoritative parent tends to be most prevalent in middle-class families, where young people's feelings are considered and the development of self-control and self-direction is valued (Baumrind, 1975). The authoritative parent retains ultimate responsibility, but is willing to discuss relevant issues, allow adolescents to voice their opinions, and work toward compromise, where possible. Authoritative parents, who are warm, accepting, and respectful of the young person's physical and pyschological privacy, enhance the young person's self-esteem and provide confidence in the possibility of affecting change and compromise through self-assertion (Coopersmith, 1967).

The Influence of Significant Adults

The ability to develop autonomy and competence is highly influenced by the relationships adolescents have with their parents. However, adolescents are also influenced by other significant adults who provide a variety of interactions from which the adolescent may make decisions on adult levels and, therefore, develop self-sufficiency and decision-making skills. Family therapists report that in cases of dysfunctional families, "community anchors" (significant adults outside the family) are particularly important to emotional development.

♦ STEREOTYPICAL ATTITUDES

In our culture, it is sometimes assumed that boys and girls will behave in certain ways because certain traits are inherent or biologically determined. More often, however, different social expectations and behaviors for males and females (as well as for students with different racial backgrounds or handicapping conditions) are learned. The evidence suggests that many stereotypes persist because they appear to be verified or because they seem desirable. For example, males may try to be rational, unemotional, ambitious, and independent because those traits are congruent with "true masculinity" or with society's ideal image of it.

Many studies have investigated how children learn their sex role identities, and social learning researchers (e.g., Mischel, 1970) believe that parents, teachers, and peers reward children for activities consistent with society's view of their gender. Maccoby and Jacklin (1974) reviewed 9,000 empirical studies and found that there is support for a biological basis for only two areas of sex differences in behavior: (1) physical aggression and dominance in males (apparently related to prenatal hormones) and (2) a female advantage in verbal skills emerging early and a male advantage in visual-spatial skills emerging at adolescence. The effect of training and learning is more important on human development than it is on other animals, and seems to modify the effects of biology. Although there may be biologically determined differences by sex, they do not preclude development of skills through environmental influences. The range of individual differences is great.

Expectations seem to play a dramatic role in the way teachers respond to students' endeavors. Representatives of minority groups or female students may sometimes be perceived by adults as "not likely to achieve" and this may, in actuality, become a self-fulfilling prophecy.

Perceptual bias refers to the influence of attitudes and values on what is actually observed (Geis, Carter, & Butler, 1982). Recognition of the fact that perceptual bias and invisible discrimination do not usually indicate conscious prejudice or ill will is often helpful. Authority figures involved with adolescents may sometimes expect them to be "difficult," and, indeed, sometimes they are! However, by reviewing the information available in the literature, we can remind ourselves of the wide range of individual differences that exist and identify aspects of behavior patterns that may trigger certain perceptual biases of our own.

The speech-language pathologist is often called upon to deal with unpredictable adolescent behavior. One way to try to understand this behavior is to identify the reasons for some adolescent coping strategies. It is probable that many students are, at times, confused about what they believe and how they should behave. Therefore, they have mixed reactions in certain situations and may exhibit negativism (e.g., saying they don't want to do something that really interests them) as a means of coping with their ambivalent mixture of excitement and anxiety.

Adolescents have difficulty maintaining continuity between the child and the emerging adult within themselves. This is demonstrated by fluctuations in levels of responsibility and reactions to disappointments, as well as by exaggerated concern for physical appearance. It is also difficult for adolescents to wrestle with the task of transforming esteemed adults from examples of perfection into ordinary people with faults and weaknesses. Many of the reactions of adolescents that adults find most perplexing are based on attempts to find coping strategies congruent with peer pressures. For the adolescent, group membership and peer acceptance is critical. The most acute difficulties for the adolescent comes from the conflict between the priorities of adults and the perspectives of the peer group.

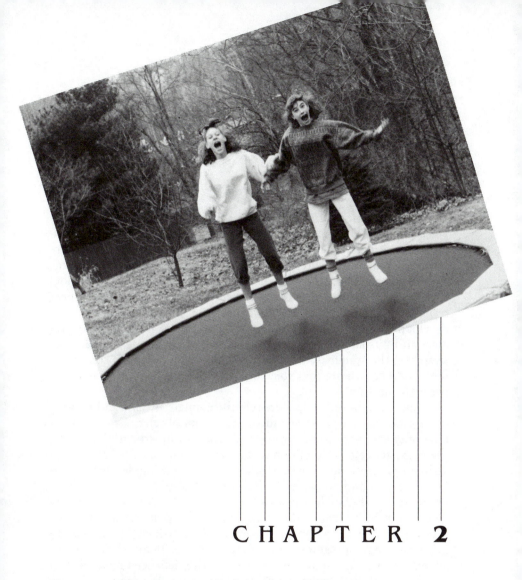

C H A P T E R **2**

Conditions that Affect Vocal Behavior During Adolescence

It is sometimes difficult to isolate the primary factor causing a voice disorder. Vocal symptoms, however, are frequently seen in conjunction with conditions that may predispose an individual to acquire a voice problem. Theoretically, any disorder (anatomical, medical, endocrinologic, psychogenic, sensory, cognitive, or muscular tension) that has the potential to alter the structure or function of the upper respiratory tract or alter affective behavior may contribute to the development of a voice disorder. Some individuals, however, may produce an unusual voice in the absence of any easily identifiable constraint on the system. Others may exhibit a whole array of conditions that could contribute to a voice disorder, but have voices that sound perfectly healthy.

Some conditions occur frequently enough in association with voice problems for clinicians to suspect a causal relationship. This is especially true with some organic and sensory impairments. However, the coexistence of a condition and a vocal symptom does not necessarily imply a relationship between the two. For example, some learning-disabled children with voice disorders also have inappropriate interpersonal skills. The cause of the voice problem in such cases may or may not be related to the interpersonal difficulties. However, the learning disability is a significant factor to be considered when designing a treatment program. The interpersonal difficulties need to be addressed since most students with voice disorders need interpersonal insight and skill to make the personal adjustments necessary to protect the vocal mechanism.

A wide variety of conditions may predispose an adolescent to develop vocal problems (see Appendix, p. 52). Frequently, many factors in combination interact to increase susceptibility to voice disorders. The adolescent years are characterized by considerable vocal activity. Both the amount and type of voice use are significant. Teenagers are typically involved in many academic, sporting, and social pursuits that involve loud talking, cheering, singing, yelling, and laughing. Telephone conversations are often protracted, emotional outbursts are intense and frequent, and group interactions often seem overexuberant to adult ears.

At the same time when the laryngeal mechanism is undergoing structural maturation, the demands upon it seem to peak. Healthy laryngeal structures, however, seem capable of withstanding a wide variety of vocal demands, although resilience of tissues in relation to severity of insult varies among individuals.

Listed below are some of the most common symptoms associated with vocal problems.

- ♦ **Hoarseness** — This symptom includes aperiodicity of fundamental frequency, random fundamental frequency variation, escape of air, and noise. Some clinicians define hoarseness as a combination of breathiness and harshness. It varies in severity and is sometimes described as mild, moderate, or severe. Hoarseness is the most prevalent symptom associated with vocal problems, and may be caused by a variety of conditions, including local and systemic diseases, disorders of motor nerves, abuse and misuse, lesions that increase size and mass of folds, inflammation, and injury.

- ♦ **Breathiness** — In a breathy voice, medial compression and longitudinal tension of the folds is lessened so that air leakage creates turbulence during vocal fold closure. The audible escape of air through lax glottal closure is perceived as aspirate noise. In its most severe form it sounds like a whisper. Lesions that effect the margins of the folds, edema, and paralysis may give rise to this symptom.

- ♦ **Harshness** — Hanley and Thurman (1970) defined harshness as an unpleasant and rough quality. There is considerable laryngeal tension and constriction and frequent hard glottal attacks. Laver and Hanson (1981) observed irregular pertubations of fundamental frequency (jitter) and intensity (shimmer).

- ♦ **Vocal fry** — Zemlin (1981) described vocal fry as being produced with the vocal folds relaxed so that the sound is emitted in discrete bursts. It is produced at the bottom of the pitch range and has been likened to the sound of popcorn popping or "creaky-door" voice.

- ♦ **Diplophonia** — This term is used to describe a "two-toned" voice or a situation in which one fold vibrates at a different rate from the other (Perkins, 1977). Some individuals can produce this at will, but in most cases it is pathological.

- ♦ **Ventricular phonation** (dysphonia plicae ventricularis) — When the false vocal folds vibrate the sound perceived is usually harsh, low pitched, and tense.

♦ **Aphonia** — This is the absence of sound during intentional phonation. It may be consistent or sporadic, acute or chronic. Time of onset may provide clues concerning etiology, e.g., upper respiratory tract infection, emotional or physical trauma, inhalation of irritants, allergic reaction, post-intubation, etc.

♦ **Syllabic aphonia** — This symptom is the absence of sound on unstressed syllables, which may occur because of difficulty adducting folds that are swollen because of allergic reactions, nodules, etc. It may occur randomly or consistently. When it occurs consistently at the ends of breath groups, syllabic aphonia may be related to inefficient use of replenishing breaths.

♦ **Dysphonia** — This disturbed phonation is perceived auditorially as breathiness, harshness, or hoarseness. Changes in normal vibratory patterns are related to size, mass, tension, or the even approximation of folds.

♦ **Hard glottal attack** — Abrupt forceful onset of phonation is frequently associated with excessive laryngeal tension and/or lack of coordination of aerodynamic and myoelastic features during initiation of phonation. It may be perceived as a grunt or click, and is frequently heard on stressed vowels in initial positions in words.

♦ **Restricted pitch range** — This may occur in the singing voice only or in speaking voice as well. It may indicate the presence of a nodule or polyp, the onset of neurological disease (e.g., myasthenia gravis), hearing loss, or a psychogenic disorder.

♦ **"Tickle" in the throat** — This symptom may be associated with dryness or strain, allergic reactions, or lesions (e.g., nodules and polyps). Swallowing may temporarily relax the tension, whereas throat clearing exacerbates it.

♦ **Dry throat** — May be related to lack of humidity and may be helped by a vaporizer at night. Mouth breathing, allergic reactions, dusty open-air environment, limited fluid intake, decongestants and antihistamines, excessive alcohol and smoking, and early diabetes may be factors.

♦ **Burning sensation in the throat** — So-called "scratchy" or "raw" throat may be caused by irritants (such as inhaled chemicals or other pollutants) or by acidic secretions from the digestive tract, as happens in hiatal hernia.

♦ **Aching throat** — Muscle tension in strap muscles of the neck may cause this, especially if the anterior part of the neck is involved. Movement of the swallowing muscles when phonating may indicate muscular hyperfunction.

♦ **Tightness in throat** — This may indicate hyperfunction, tension in pharyngeal muscles, retracted tongue position, or edema of vocal folds (e.g., allergic reaction).

♦ **Lump in throat** — This sensation can occur in association with extreme stress, hiatal hernia, or thyroid enlargement.

♦ **Pain** — Disorders of the temporomandibular joint, contact ulcers, intubation, trauma, prolonged vocal abuse, inflammatory conditions, or referred pain from the ear may cause complaints.

♦ **Mucus strand** — A strand of mucus at the junction of the anterior and mid-third portions of the folds may be noted during laryngeal examination. It seems to appear at the point of maximum excursion of the folds and is associated with nodule and polyp formation and with vocal abuse and strain.

♦ **Fatigue after voice use** — Vocal abuse, polyps and neoplasms (rare in adolescence), early paresis, and neurological disease may cause this symptom. "Vocal endurance" may be measured in a diagnostic session.

♦ **Throat clearing** — Throat clearing may be (1) an attempt to clear secretions related to allergic conditions, (2) a nervous habit or "starter", (3) the residual of an earlier respiratory tract problem now resolved, (4) related to a hiatal hernia. Frequently the individual does not realize that throat clearing has become habitual.

♦ **Inappropriate pitch variability** — When an individual uses limited pitch variability it may be due to sensory deficits (e.g., hearing loss), intellectual impairment, depression or paralysis of folds. Occasionally lesions of the folds may also preclude the use of higher pitches (because of increased size and mass), thus affecting general pitch variability. Sometimes, too, a vocal abuser may restrict voice change to loudness changes. In such cases it may be beneficial to teach the abuser some other methods of varying the voice.

♦ **Inappropriately high pitch level** — An abnormally high pitch for age and sex may be related to delayed or incongruous pubertal development, a small web, mutational falsetto, or learned behavior.

♦ **Inappropriately low pitch level** — An abnormally low pitch may be habituated through choice by some individuals who prefer a "deep" or "throaty" voice. A person's "vocal image" (Cooper, 1973) may need to be explored. Other factors to be considered include contact ulcers, virilization, edema, tumors, nodules (or any lesion increasing size and mass of folds) or paralysis that decreases elasticity of folds.

◆ **Weak volume level** — A weak or thin voice may be due to respiratory limitations, lack of resonance, reduced valving capacity of larynx or psychosocial factors.

It is useful to review conditions that heighten an adolescent's susceptibility to voice problems and to identify constraints on the voice system that may influence etiology, maintenance of disorders, and treatment. Therapy programs will be designed more appropriately and implemented more effectively if all pertinent factors have been considered. Recognizing factors that can trigger behavioral compensations helps a speech-language pathologist to identify the behaviors and to help students recognize and extinguish or shape these behaviors.

The vulnerability of the laryngeal structures to abuse and misuse seems to be heightened by factors that irritate the mucosa. Irritated tissues react more readily to insult, and chronic irritation in combination with chronic vocal abuse is particularly significant in the etiology of voice disorders. An individual with irritated and swollen folds often adopts compensatory vocal practices (e.g., forceful adduction, louder level, throat clearing) that exacerbate the original problem. An overlay of secondary abusive practices may be misguided attempts to compensate for structural changes that were caused by primary irritants.

◆ *SORE THROAT*

Sore throat is a symptom of many different illnesses, and its cause may be hard to diagnose. Illnesses responsible for sore throats may be as serious as leukemia or as relatively harmless as a common cold.

The upper respiratory tract is lined with mucous membrane, which feels moist and slippery (the inside of the mouth is lined with mucous membrane). Infections, allergic reactions, and irritation can cause inflammation of these tissues. Infections that can cause sore throats may be bacterial, viral, or fungal. Fungal infections are the least common causes of sore throat, and viral infections are the most common causes (the common cold is caused by a virus). A sore throat is usually accompanied by a runny nose and a generally miserable feeling. Since antibiotics are not used to treat viral infections, a physician usually recommends rest (to help the body fight infection), fluids (to keep tissues moist and to thin mucus secretions so they can be expelled), and aspirin (to reduce feelings of discomfort).

Bacterial infections, on the other hand, are usually treated with antibiotics prescribed by a physician. An example of a bacterial infection is strep throat, which is caused by streptococcal germs. Symptoms of strep throat include fever, white or yellow spots on the throat lining, and pain when swallowing. The illness is potentially dangerous because it may lead to rheumatic fever or to kidney infection if not accurately diagnosed and treated by a physician. The only accurate way to diagnose strep throat is by taking a throat culture.

Tonsillitis is another common cause of sore throat and may be due to either viral or bacterial infection. It is a painful inflammation of the tonsils, bulges of lymph tissue on either side of the back of the mouth. Although it is not known why, these infections most often occur in children aged 3 to 7 and 12 to 13. However, adults who still have their tonsils may also suffer from tonsillitis. Forty years ago, tonsillectomies were recommended by physicians for almost all children. Today, however, the operation is recommended only when there is a high frequency of recurrence (e.g., four to seven episodes per year) or when the tonsils are so swollen that breathing is affected. Another viral illness, mononucleosis, often strikes teenagers and adults and causes uncomfortable sore throat and other debiliitating symptoms.

Allergies can cause sore throat if the sufferer is allergic to airborne substances (such as dust, pollen, animal dander, or mold) or ingested substances that cause changes in the upper respiratory tract (such as foods or drugs that affect tissues lining the tract). Excessive dryness or overproduction of secretions are typical reactions to allergens. Sometimes an allergic condition may be exacerbated by a secondary infection or by overuse of an irritated mechanism.

Irritation of the delicate tissues of the throat may also be caused by smoking, drinking alcohol (which results in dryness of the tissues), and by digestive problems, which can result in the backing-up of stomach contents into the esophagus and pharynx. Reflux of acids may occur at night, when an individual is lying down, and may be responsible for chronic morning sore throat. Antacids can often soothe sore throats caused by stomach acids. Some clinical evidence suggests that repeated vomiting (such as in girls with bulimia) can be damaging to throat tissues.

Sore throats often seem more prevalent during winter months, when people tend to congregate indoors. Since infectious agents may be spread by air and touch, it is important to wash hands frequently and to avoid rubbing the eyes and nose or touching the mouth. Good nutrition and adequate rest also help the body resist infection. A dry atmosphere, without adequate humidity, dries out throat membranes, and nasal stuffiness increases mouth breathing. Since dryness increases susceptibility to infection, drinking liquids and using a humidifier are frequently helpful. People who are susceptible to allergies should check for molds and fungi in damp basements, and on objects such as plants, books, and shower curtains. Dust-harboring objects should be removed from sleeping areas, and the head should be elevated during sleep. Inhalation of steam may also help dislodge excess mucus.

If a sore throat is the result of a cold, a visit to a physician is probably not necessary. However, a doctor should be consulted if there is a possibility of strep throat or if a sore throat is accompanied by difficulty in breathing, earache, rash, fever greater than 103°F, inability to swallow saliva, and difficulty opening the mouth. If a sore throat has not gone away within two or three weeks, an appointment with an otolaryngologist (ear, nose, and throat specialist) is recommended.

◆ ASTHMA

Symptoms of asthma include shortness of breath, wheezing, and the production of excess mucus in the passages leading to the lungs. Attacks can be terrifying if the patient cannot breathe easily. Exhalation is usually affected by obstructed or constricted airways. Asthma attacks may be triggered by respiratory infections, cold air, exercise, allergens such as pollens, and molds, chemicals, and pollutants. Occasionally, the attacks may be exacerbated by emotional upset.

Treatment of Asthma

Histamine is a chemical in the body that is released in response to allergens if a person's immune system is extra-sensitive to a substance. Histamine causes blood vessels to dilate and leak fluids, which cause tissues to become red and itchy. Antihistamines are drugs that slow down the action of histamine and help control allergic symptoms. Oral decongestants are used in association with antihistamines. Decongestants reduce fluid build-up and ease nasal congestion. Allergy shots are sometimes prescribed to desensitize the immune system to specific allergens. Nebulizers and sprays are also used to treat asthma and allergy symptoms. It is best to seek medical advice rather than to use nonprescription medications for persistent symptoms involving the ears, nose, throat, or breathing system.

◆ ALLERGIES

The National Instititue of Allergies and Infectious Diseases (Joseph & Mills, 1983) estimate that approximately 31 million Americans (i.e., 15 out of every 100 persons) suffer from one or more significant allergies. The same percentage applies in Canada. This is probably a conservative estimate. Allergies are responsible for more than 36 million school days lost by children in the United States every year. Because allergic reactions are manifested in so many different ways, they are frequently misdiagnosed and untreated.

Allergy may be defined as a condition of unusual sensitivity to foreign substances or environmental conditions. The substance an individual is allergic to is known as an allergen or antigen. Allergens may be inhaled, digested, touched, or injected, and responses to them vary. Inhaling a certain substance could produce a rash in one person, whereas eating the same substance could produce breathing difficulties in another. Reactions to allergens may be immediate or delayed. Hives, bronchial asthma, hay fever, drug reactions, and reactions to insect bites are usually apparent immediately after exposure, whereas skin reactions to chemicals (e.g., poison ivy or cosmetics) and diarrhea are delayed.

When an allergen such as pollen enters blood vessels in the lining of the nose, a variety of allergic reactions may take place in the vocal tract. The muscles surrounding breathing passages contract and cause spasms that restrict air flow. Additionally, large amounts of mucus may be discharged into the air tubes, which further hinders free breathing. Dilation of blood vessels causes swelling in adjoining tissues lining nasal cavities and bronchial tubes.

Allergens in combination appear to have a cumulative effect. If, for example, an individual is exposed to two allergens simultaneously (e.g., inhaling pollen and eating nuts), the interaction of the two allergens may result in an allergic response that would not occur if the exposure was limited to only one of the substances.

It is common for allergic patterns to change at puberty. Sometimes manifestations take different forms or disappear during adolescence. Some girls, for example, experience relief from asthma when they begin to menstruate. In other cases, adolescence may be a time when allergic symptoms are noted for the first time. The onset of hypersensitivity to weeds, grasses, trees, or mold spores may be associated with relocation to a different geographic area or may be related to increased outdoor activity. Seasonal variations may also affect symptoms. For example, molds are parasitic plants that grow on corn, wheat, and oats, and mold spores are blown through the air during the summer, especially in grain-growing regions. Molds are also found in stored grain, straw, and hay. Unlike the pollens from weeds and grasses, spores are not killed by freezing weather. Perennial allergic rhinitis (inflammation of the mucous membranes of the nose) occurs year round from unseasonal substances such as mold (on houseplants, in paper products, in damp basements), house dust, and animal dander. Seasonal rhinitis (e.g., ragweed) is more transitory, depending on pollinating seasons in various areas. Weather may exacerbate allergic reactions (e.g., cool rainy days or humid conditions may increase the effects of molds and chemical pollutants in the air), and hot, sunny, windy conditions may alleviate suffering temporarily.

Drug allergies are particularly important in relation to the adolescent population. Drugs may be sniffed, sprayed, rubbed on the skin, or taken orally or by injection. Tranquilizers, aspirin, and a variety of "recreational" drugs cause adverse allergic effects in some individuals. Penicillin is well known as a drug that can be potentially life-threatening to some sensitive people. Nonprescription drugs, however, pose the greatest threat to adolescents. Allergic reactions to drugs range from mild rashes to death, and include hives, wheezing, sneezing, swelling of lips and tongue, pain from an inflamed intestinal tract, dizziness from circulatory disturbances, and pallor related to anemia. The lymph nodes may enlarge, the kidneys may slow down, and the heart may become inflamed. A distorted response to medication may include a lowering of the white blood cell count, resulting in a lowered resistance to infection. Liver damage may also occur with prolonged drug use (Joseph & Mills, 1983).

Treatment of Allergies

Since respiration and phonation, and thus, the quality of an individual's voice, can be greatly affected by allergic reactions, a speech-language pathologist should carefully explore with the student the possibility of unidentified allergies. It is not unusual for a therapy plan to consist of environmental and medical control of allergy in conjunction with a program of vocal hygiene. A vocal hygiene program is important for teaching a student ways to avoid stressing an already "at risk" mechanism.

Antihistamines may be used to control hay fever or upper respiratory tract problems. They are given orally or injected. The "drying" effect of antihistamines is useful in controlling symptoms such as sneezing and runny nose. Antihistamines are never recommended for an asthmatic because they hamper the ability to cough up sputum and intensify the asthmatic's difficulties. One side effect of antihistamines includes loss of alertness. Coordination problems may occur when antihistamines are combined with decongestants. Students who use antihistamines to alleviate nasal secretions may also suffer from dryness throughout the laryngeal mucosa. Excessively dry tissues are particularly at risk for vocal abuse.

Desensitizing injections are used to treat severe allergic reactions, particularly to pollen and molds. This treatment, of course, requires expert medical consultation. Very severe allergic conditions, and especially incapacitating asthma attacks, are treated with hormone drugs (e.g., cortisone), but physicians use these cautiously since the side effects are sometimes quite dangerous.

♦ CHEMICALLY INDUCED IRRITATION

Individuals vary in their reactions to chemical substances. For example, some people are highly sensitive to cigarette smoke, whereas others are barely affected by it. The possibility for irritation of tissues from smoke inhalation should be considered during the diagnostic process since many middle and high school students smoke cigarettes. Mouth washes and gargles, if used excessively, can also cause mucosal irritation. Gastro-esophageal reflux has been identified as causing severe dental, pharyngeal, and laryngeal irritation in adolescents who are bulimic (especially girls). However, mild reflux may occur in many individuals during sleep. The inhalation of noxious fumes, either intentionally or because of environmental pollution, also occurs with deleterious effects on the laryngeal structures of some adolescents. Sometimes exposure to industrial pollution or dust results in excessive dryness of the respiratory tract, and this lack of lubrication creates a high-risk environment for vocal abuse (Punt, 1979). Similarly, however, exposure to air-borne irritants can cause excessive mucus to be produced in the tract, and postnasal drip and laryngeal secretions can lead to increased frequency of abusive throat clearing and coughing. Over-the-counter medications, such as antihistamines and decongestants, are sometimes used excessively by teenagers who are trying to control high levels of vocal tract congestion. Pharmacologically induced dryness can occur as a result. Recreational drugs and birth control pills may cause swelling of the nasal or laryngeal mucosa.

A speech-language pathologist should obtain a complete history of exposure to chemical agents during voice evaluation. Since most adolescents are reluctant to provide specific information, the speech-language pathologist should word questions concerning drug use in a nonjudgmental way: "How often do you use _____?" "Which of the following best fits *your* pattern of smoking? More than a pack a day, a pack a day, less than a pack a day." "Have you noticed an increase in nasal congestion with some drugs more than others?"

♦ VOCALLY DEMANDING ACTIVITIES

The type and amount of vocalization and the vocal adjustments the individual makes during sustained vocalization, especially against background noise, are significant with respect to susceptibility to voice disorders. Susceptibility may also be affected by the individual's general level of health and fatigue.

Types of extracurricular activities, the balance between quiet and noisy activities, and the manner of voice production during sustained or projected vocalization are important considerations when evaluating predisposition toward voice problems. Many factors interrelate in placing an individual "at risk." For example, the student who sings a great deal but uses voice inappropriately is obviously more vulnerable than one who naturally uses an appropriate technique or is studying with a qualified voice teacher. Members of athletic teams whose voices are used constantly in the open air, students who abuse alcohol and engage in rowdy parties, and character actors who use a variety of distorted phonatory patterns may run the risk of subjecting their mechanisms to unusual levels of stress.

Jensen (1964) found that 12 percent of 377 high school cheerleaders studied had hoarse voice quality. Andrews and Shank (1983) studied 102 females aged 13 to 17 years and found that 37 percent reported a history of voice problems. Older girls with more years of cheerleading experience reported more voice difficulties than did girls with less cheerleading experience. In a questionnaire (Reich, McHenry, & Keaton, 1986) administered to 146 cheerleaders, it was found that episodes of "tired voice" and "sore throat" increased significantly following cheerleading events. The evidence suggests that both acute and chronic laryngeal changes (aphonia, aphonic syllables, diplophonia, and pitch breaks) occur more frequently among cheerleaders than among noncheerleaders.

♦ RESPIRATORY DISORDERS

Any condition that makes it difficult for a student to inhale deeply, or to prolong and control the exhalation phase of speech breathing, can limit vocal performance. Tracheal stenosis (narrowing of the airway) or pulmonary obstruction is usually significant in these cases. Stenosis of subglottal structures frequently results from birth defects, trauma, inflammatory conditions, or intubation injuries and their sequelae. Severe problems (e.g., congenital malformations) are usually identified early in life and are not likely to be seen in untreated form in teenagers. Mild-to-moderate stenosis may occur for a variety of reasons, and is usually characterized by stridor with deep and rapid breathing, especially during exercise and physical exertion. Dyspnea during exertion, cough, or intermittent wheezing related to excessive or thickened secretions may also be observed and, occasionally, misdiagnosed as asthma. In asthma, constriction and spasms of the airway generally cause wheezing only during the exhalation phase of breathing.

Sleep apnea, the transient cessation of breathing during sleeping, affects some adolescents. Tonsillar tissue and craniofacial anomalies (e.g., Treacher Collins syndrome, Stickler syndrome, hemifacial microsmia) may make individuals prone of obstructive sleep apnea (Sher et al., 1985). Micronathia (e.g., Pierre Robin syndrome) seems to heighten the risk of sleep apnea because the tongue moves back and blocks the pharyngeal cavity during sleep. Symptoms that may be associated with sleep apnea include snoring, restless sleep, interrupted respiration cycles during sleep, fluctuations in weight, hyperactive gag reflex, and speech problems. Obstructive sleep apnea does not have a direct effect on the voice; however, it may occur together with mouth breathing, resulting in dry mucosal tissues and hoarseness.

Respiratory obstruction and/or excessive secretions result in coughing that may also irritate laryngeal mucosa. Many serious illnesses (e.g., cystic fibrosis), inflammatory conditions (e.g., infections, allergies), growths (e.g., papillomatosis of the bronchi or trachea), and systemic diseases may limit respiratory function. Obesity may also contribute to some respiratory difficulties. The checklist in Table 2-1 (which is certainly not exhaustive) may be helpful during history-taking.

TABLE 2-1.
Respiratory Conditions Affecting
Breathing Efficiency

Paresis/paralysis of respiratory muscles
Congenital abnormalities
Trauma/stenosis
Tracheal amyloidosis
Broncheal/tracheal papillomatosis
Immotile cilia syndrome
Chronic infections (e.g., bronchitis)
Asthma
Allergies
Smoke inhalation/pollution
Iatrogenic respiratory disease
Chemical reactions (e.g., drugs, alcohol)
Cystic fibrosis
Foreign bodies
Obstructive sleep apnea
Tumor

TABLE 2-2.
Exercising Breathing Muscles

1. Place hands on sides of lower chest.
2. Breathe in slowly, observing movement of the lower chest.
3. Keep shoulders and upper chest relaxed.
4. Breath out slowly through pursed lips, trying to extend the length of the exhalation and timing each successive trial.
5. Practice several times a day and rest or hold breath if dizziness occurs.

Treatment of Respiratory Disorders

Exercise is helpful for some types of respiratory disease. Physicians, physical therapists and respiratory therapists frequently provide guidelines for individuals with chronic respiratory problems, and a speech-language pathologist should never implement a program of breathing exercises (Table 2-2) before obtaining appropriate information concerning medical status. The following suggestions, however, may be useful with some students. Students who complain of breathlessness should be encouraged to relax, breathe in slowly, and purse the lips in a whistling position and blow out slowly and evenly, attempting to increase the length of the exhalation phase. Pursed-lip breathing may be used whenever a student feels short of breath. It should be explained to students that this technique maintains air pressure in the airway so that more stale air can be breathed out. Sometimes clogged or narrowed airways or damaged air sacs in the lungs trap stale air.

Coughing spells are frightening, embarrassing, and tiring. The cough reflex is useful when it expels mucus and clears the airway. Productive coughing (Table 2-3) comes from deep in the lungs, and students may need to be taught the difference between a cough that expels mucus and one that is nonproductive. A nonproductive

TABLE 2-3.
Controlled Coughing

1. Sit in a chair with feet on floor and head slightly forward.
2. Take a deep breath.
3. Hold breath for a few seconds.
4. Cough twice (once to loosen mucus and once to bring it up).
5. Breath in by sniffing gently.
6. Spit out the mucus into tissue (do not swallow mucus as this can upset the stomach).

cough may be habituated and cause unnecessary irritation of laryngeal structures.

When dryness is a problem, it is important that students increase fluid intake (usually eight glasses of water a day) and use humidifiers or vaporizers to moisturize the air. Fluids and moisturized air help to soften mucus so that it can be more easily expectorated. However, humidifiers and vaporizers must be carefully cleaned on a regular basis because they can harbor and breed germs. Sometimes postural drainage is recommended to help drain mucus from the lungs. Postural drainage (Table 2-4) tilts the body so that mucus moves from the lungs into the upper airway where it is more easily expelled. (There are many possible positions, and a physician will usually recommend one that is appropriate for the individual.)

Medications

Physicians may prescribe medications for people with respiratory disease. The speech-language pathologist should ask about medica-

TABLE 2-4.
Exercises and Positions to Open Airways

Postural Drainage*

♦ Place a pillow under the hips (so that chest is lower) and lie prone on the floor, or lie on back with pillow under hips and knees raised.
♦ Clap or vibrate the chest to help loosen mucus.

Other Postural Exercises to Open Airway

♦ Raise arms during inhalation and lower arms during exhalation.
♦ Sit in a straight chair with shoulders relaxed and breathe in. During exhalation, turn trunk to left, reach arms over left shoulder, and bounce. Repeat on right side.
♦ Lie down, place hands behind head, and breathe in. Breathe out while raising head and shoulders as high as possible. Feel the stomach muscles tighten, but don't sit up completely.
♦ Lie down and raise the right knee toward chest while breathing out. Breathe in as leg is lowered. Repeat with left knee and then both knees. Switch and breathe in while raising knees and breathe out while lowering them.
♦ Lie down and tilt pelvis during deep breathing. Relax during inspiration. Tighten muscles of stomach and buttocks during expiration.
♦ Sit in a chair, lean back, and raise arms during inspiration. Then lean forward slowly until chest lies on legs and head falls to knees (chin tucked under chest). Exhale slowly, feeling the movement on legs.

*Often best when done early in the morning to clear mucus that has built up during the night. In the evening it should be done at least an hour before bedtime.

tions that adolescents may be using on doctor's orders, as well as those they may be taking without medical advice.

◆ *Bronchodilators* come in various forms, including pills, liquids, and sprays. Side effects include insomnia, nervousness, and upset stomach.

◆ *Nebulizers* are sprayers that deliver a mist that can be breathed into the lungs. They should be used carefully under a doctor's direction.

◆ *Expectorants* are used to make mucus thinner and easier to expel.

◆ *Sedatives and tranquilizers* are occasionally prescribed to promote relaxation or to help a person sleep. However, they can dangerously slow breathing if too many are taken.

◆ *Steroids* are strong medications that are sometimes prescribed to reduce swelling in the airways and to ease breathing. They also increase energy. If used for a long time, steroids can have the following side effects: fullness in the face, stomach ulcers, weakened skin and bones, tendency to bruise easily, and decreased immunity to infection. Since they slow down the adrenal glands, they must be tapered off gradually.

◆ *Antibiotics* are used only for treating bacterial infections since viruses do not respond to them. Side effects include stomach upset and skin rashes.

◆ *Diuretics* are sometimes called "water pills" and are used to rid the body of extra fluid. Reduced salt intake is also recommended in such cases. Use of diuretics is linked to potassium loss, which can cause weakness and muscle cramps.

◆ PHONATION

Any change in tissue that interferes with vocal fold approximation, equal distribution of vocal fold weight, size or mass may disturb normal laryngeal vibration.

By the time students reach the middle and high school years, most congenital anomalies of the laryngeal structures have been identified. However, small laryngeal webs are occasionally undetected prior to puberty if they do not significantly obstruct the airway. (The majority of congenital laryngeal webs occur at the vocal fold level and only approximately 25 percent occur in the supraglottal and infraglottal areas.) In the case of a small web, the voice of a prepubertal child may not sound significantly different from those of peers. However, at the time of vocal mutation, when the peer group demonstrates more mature vocal characteristics, a higher-pitched voice, for example, may finally draw attention to a student with a small web. Students who have been treated surgically for removal of webs during infancy may occasionally demonstrate residual effects of earlier intervention during later life. Careful history-taking is critical in order to identify vocal symptoms related to early trauma, surgeries and intubation. Questions concerning any conditions related to airway obstruction, for example, should routinely be asked when the speech pathologist interviews students and parents.

Some teenagers who had multiple surgeries for papillomatosis as children may exhibit hoarseness, compensatory hyperfunctional vocal behavior, or overly protective vocal patterns such as extreme breathiness and minimal loudness. Laryngeal edema and posterior commissure narrowing may occur as a result of previous intubation. Postsurgically, patients often use the same pattern of laryngeal control that they developed to compensate for lesions before surgery. Scar tissue at the site of a lesion may reduce the pliable mucosal covering and, therefore, the vibration at that part of the fold. Iatrogenic injury subsequent to surgical removal of benign lesions near the anterior commissure may also result in web formation.

Penetrating neck trauma may sometimes result in hematoma that compresses the airway and produces symptoms of stridor and dysphonia. Trauma may also result in lacerated mucosa, fractured cartilage, or displaced arytenoids. Signs of laryngeal trauma include palpable fracture, stridor, dyspnea, dysphagia, laryngeal pain or tenderness, hemoptysis, hoarseness, and aphonia/dysphonia.

Systemic diseases, such as leukemia and anemia, and infectious diseases, such as diphtheria, may affect laryngeal function, and are frequently associated with lowered resistance to respiratory tract infections. Endocrine disorders (e.g., thyroid dysfunction) may produce symptoms of hoarseness, as can nodules, polyps, papilloma, and hyperkeratosis. Benign neoplasms (neurofibromas, hemangiomas, lymphangiomas), cysts, and laryngoceles may occur infrequently and disrupt phonation, depending on the site of the lesion. Ulcers and granulomas sometimes occur and are thought to be residuals of intubation trauma.

Occasionally, an acute episode of hoarseness may be triggered in a healthy larynx by excessive vocal abuse, such as cheering for prolonged periods of time. More common, however, is chronic hoarseness that results from vocal abuse in association with other factors that irritate tissues in the airway and, specifically, in the larynx. Irritated (i.e., red or swollen) folds are particularly susceptible to long periods of use, misuse, sudden overexertion, and compensatory attempts at forceful adduction. Allergic reactions affecting the mucous membranes of the fold frequently result in inflammation and edema. Approximation of the folds is inhibited and vocal fold vibration is impaired.

Vocal Pathologies

Vocal nodules are small noncancerous growths that occur on the vocal folds. They are caused by irritation of the delicate membranes covering the muscles, and are one of the most common disorders of the larynx. Nodules appear as small bumps on the vibrating edge of one or both folds. Since "lateral" means "side," they are described as "unilateral" if there is only one, and "bilateral" if they occur on both sides (i.e., one on each of the vocal folds). When the vocal folds come together during speaking or singing, the free edges of the folds must approximate evenly for a clear voice to be produced. When vocal nodules are present, the folds are unable to meet evenly along their entire length and leakage of air occurs when voice is produced. The weight of the nodules may also cause the vocal folds to vibrate unevenly during voice production, causing diplophonia. People with vocal nodules speak with a hoarse voice quality. Other symptoms of vocal nodules include voice breaks, restricted pitch range, lower pitch level, and observable tension in the muscles of the neck. When nodules are small, the voice may sound clearest when a person is speaking loudly or on a high pitch. Throat clearing and coughing may also be noted. Treatments include surgery, voice rest, and the elimination of abusive vocal practices. Speech-language therapy to encourage appropriate vocal hygiene and nonstressful vocal production is recommended so that nodules do not recur.

Vocal nodules, polyps, and hyperkeratosis are frequently seen in "performance-oriented" young adults. Among singers, nodules seem most common in sopranos (Punt, 1979; Brodnitz, 1971). Young adults, particularly females, who are talkative or active in dramatics, musicals, cheerleading, or other peformance-related activities seem especially susceptible to developing nodules.

Signs of vocal pathology include lack of stability of vocal behaviors and atypical pitch range, loudness, or quality. Pitch level is considered in relation to age, sex, and pubertal development. Judgments of appropriateness of pitch levels can be correlated with acoustic measures. Perkins (1977) found that in nine studies 27 different terms were used to describe quality defects. This illustrates one of the problems of describing quality in perceptual terms. However, individuals with sudden onset of voice problems usually report that their voices have changed significantly. When quality deviations cause an adolescent embarrassment or frustration, the problem is real, despite professional difficulty with descriptive terminology. A weak voice, in which loudness cannot be sustained without difficulty, frequently causes fatigue from the strain of talking. Hyperfunctional muscle involvement is a common compensation in such cases and may compound the original problem. Problems of organic etiology are frequently characterized by difficulties with appropriate loudness. Sometimes an individual with vocal nodules can produce a clear voice only when speaking loudly. By over-adducting the folds, the effect of the lesion is minimized until the nodules increase significantly in size. Speaking loudly or at a higher pitch to "clear" the voice quality is not an effective long-term strategy. This hyperfunctional pattern exacerbates the lesion further. Excessive throat clearing, a strategy used by some speakers with conditions that increase the size and mass of the folds, is also detrimental. Usually it is more sensible to substitute swallowing for throat clearing.

The fact that such a variety of medical problems may be accompanied by hoarseness underscores the need for medical referral and evaluation of teenagers who exhibit chronically hoarse voices. A speech-language pathologist should be vigilant in ensuring that students and parents are alerted to the importance of a medical examination in diagnosis and management. In fact, a medical report prior to the initiation of voice therapy is required by most speech-language pathologists. Table 2-5 is a list of suggestions for decreasing vocal strain.

Mutational Falsetto

If a male has completed the process of puberty (i.e., genital growth, skeletal growth, and secondary sex changes) but maintains a childlike vocal pattern, the condition is called *mutational falsetto.* Medical examination is necessary to ensure that endocrinologic or structural problems are not present. Greene (1972) said that the larynx is usually pulled up high in the throat and the musculature is tense. Frequently, demonstration of the availability of a lower pitch results in habituation of more adult pitch levels. Partial mutation may be observed in some boys. Aronson (1973) described voice therapy for mutational falsetto and stressed the need to ensure that a boy is com-

TABLE 2-5.
Ways to Decrease Vocal Strain

◆ Use nonverbal "attention getters" such as clapping, waving, and hand signals rather than the voice whenever possible.
◆ Make use of "mouthing" during unison singing or cheering.
◆ Increase listening time and quiet activities.
◆ Reduce the distance between yourself and the listener so there will be no need to shout.
◆ Avoid hard glottal attacks when you speak.
◆ Maintain good posture and relax your neck, jaw, and shoulders.
◆ Avoid repeated throat clearing and nonproductive coughing.
◆ Avoid talking in the presence of loud noise.
◆ Avoid talking during periods of upper respiratory problems.
◆ Avoid smoking.
◆ Drink lots of water to improve lubrication of the throat.
◆ Learn to be a good questioner and encourage others to talk. Increase the ratio of listening versus talking.
◆ Use pitch and rate changes rather than loudness changes in order to get and hold attention.
◆ Always use plenty of air when you speak and breathe frequently.

---

fortable with his newly acquired voice. Many clinicians have hypothesized that the retention of a high-pitched voice by a postpubertal male is related to underlying psychosocial conflicts and that psychological counseling may be needed (Aronson, 1973). Wilson (1987) noted that an effective test for mutational falsetto is to ask a boy to breathe deeply and to cough or say a vowel with an abrupt glottal attack. Other techniques include using other vegetative functions such as sighing or laughing. Gutzman's pressure tests (Luchsinger & Arnold, 1965) or other digital manipulations of the larynx may be used to demonstrate the availability of a lower pitch level. Symptoms associated with mutational falsetto include high pitch level, pitch breaks, minimal vocal variety, thin breathy or hoarse quality, shallow breathing, muscle tension, reduced loudness, and reticence and embarrassment in conversational interactions.

Speech-language pathologists should also be aware that an apparent absence of pubertal vocal change may be related to a nutritional or medical problem delaying puberty. Undernutrition due to anorexia nervosa or bulimia (primarily in girls), a systemic disease resulting in malabsorption of nutrients, and obesity can all inhibit puberty. Maturational delays may also be caused by collagen diseases, anemias, cardiac disorders, severe renal disesases, and diseases of the respiratory tract. When questions concerning pubertal development occur, medical evaluation is warranted.

♦ *RESONANCE*

Craniofacial anomalies of serious proportion are usually identified during childhood and are rarely encountered in the teenage population without a treatment history. When a severe organic abnormality is present, a medical history is usually available for the speech-language pathologist. Sequelae of earlier trauma (e.g., scar tissue, reconstructive procedures, and surgical aftermaths) occasionally present unusual symptoms during adolescence, but again case history information can generally be obtained and current symptoms can be analyzed with respect to pertinent medical information. A speech-language pathologist may also need to obtain information from orthodontists, since many adolescents receive orthodontic treatment.

Acute pharyngitis refers to all acute infections of the pharynx, including the tonsils and adenoids. Systemic diseases that cause pharyngitis include infectious hepatitis, toxoplasmosis, infectious mononucleosis, and herpangina. Infectious mononucleosis is a viral disease that frequently occurs in teenagers. Although rarely life threatening, "mono" causes extreme fatigue and discomfort in swallowing and can recur. Occasionally a teenager may also contract a fungal infection affecting the upper respiratory tract, but this is much less common than bacterial or viral infections. Occasionally, a lateral pharyngeal abcess occurs during adolescence. Generally, speech-language pathologists are not concerned with acute conditions due to infection. It is chronic conditions that tend to be related to voice problems.

Chronic rhinitis and chronic sinusitis may create symptoms of hyponasality because of partial or complete nasal obstruction. Nasal polyps and septal defects may also cause hyponasality. Hyponasality (also called "denasality") is perceived as "blocked nose" voice. Any obstruction (partial or complete) of the nasal cavities may cause this resonance pattern. In adolescents, sports injuries, allergic rhinitis, chronic sinusitis, growths, adenoiditis, premenstrual edema of nasal mucosa, and drug use (e.g., cocaine) should be considered as causes of hyponasality. Habitual mouth breathing, often in association with dryness of laryngeal structures, is frequently seen.

The tonsils and adenoids regress during adolescence, but episodes of adenotonsillitis are frequent and occasionally occur as part of systemic diseases, such as gonorrhea and immunodeficiencies. Neoplasms of the nose and paranasal sinuses may also occur and show symptoms of hyponasality. Angiofibromas occur in adolescent males. These are vascular lesions occurring in the posterior nasal or nasopharyngeal areas.

Trauma to the face may result in frontal sinus fracture, nasal septum damage, or maxillary, mandibular, or soft tissue injury. Residuals of past trauma may affect mouth opening, the resonating cavities, and neurological function. Penetrating wounds to the skull base, for example, may affect both the glossopharyngeal and vagus nerves, resulting in both dysphagia and vocal fold paralysis. Handler and Wetmore (1982) described sports-related injuries that can occur in childhood and adolescence and advocated the use of protective masks.

Videofluoroscopy and flexible fiber-optic nasopharyngoscopy techniques have made it possible for clinicians to observe movement of the velopharyngeal sphincter during speech. Such studies yield valuable information concerning function of the sphincter and changes with age. Sadewitz and Shprintzen (1985) found significant change in the morphology of the oropharynx and nasopharynx. As children develop through adolescence, the relationship of the velum to the pharynx changes, producing a shift in angulation of the orifice. The relative anterioposterior dimensions of the velopharyngeal movement had decreased in most of Sadewitz and Shprintzen's subjects who were retested after ten years. The actual point at which the velum contacted the pharyngeal wall had changed in all subjects, and the relationship between the planes of lateral wall movement and velar elevation had also changed. Passavant's pad was present in only two subjects when the original testing occurred in childhood, but was present in five subjects when retesting occurred during the teenage years.

Children with obstructed airways due to enlarged tonsils or adenoids frequently have trouble eating because they are mouth breathers. Thus, they eat slowly and eat less. Removal of the lymphatic tissue results in improved eating habits and weight gain (Pasquariello et al., 1985). However, removal of tonsils and adenoids in the presence of velopharyngeal insufficiency and/or submucous clefts can result in symptoms of hypernasality and nasal emission. Hypernasality may be observed in adolescents with normal velopharyngeal mechanisms for about six weeks following removal of tonsils and adenoids. This is a temporary condition related to learning new speech and voice patterns with an altered mechanism.

Hypernasality, sometimes called "nasal" voice, may be accompanied by nasal emission and incorrect production of consonants requiring oral breath pressure (e.g., if velopharyngeal inadequacy is present). Hypernasality that is inconsistent, especially when it occurs only when the system is fatigued, is considered a possible early sign of neurological disease (e.g., myasthenia gravis or multiple sclerosis). When hypernasality occurs only on vowels, it may be referred to as "assimilated" nasality and may be due to the influence of nasal consonants (e.g., pãn). Word pairs such as (pat, pan) can be used to ascertain whether nasal production of the vowel is indeed the result of the adjacent nasal consonant. Nasal production of vowel sounds is frequent in some regional speech patterns (e.g., Indiãna) and may be due to faulty learning, or may be habituated as a result of certain emotional states (e.g., whining). It is not usually considered a problem unless an individual aspires to professional use of voice (e.g., broadcasting, acting, singing).

Postsurgical alterations in the vocal tract (e.g., repaired clefts, secondary procedures such as pharyngeal flaps, reduced tissue subsequent to tonsillectomy and adenoidectomy, and scar tissue) should be documented through interviews, histories, and medical reports. Compensatory behaviors may be intricately related to such alterations. A mixed pattern of both hypernasality and hyponasality may be present.

Faulty learning, regional dialects, and psychosocial factors may also affect the development and maintenance of appropriate resonance behavior. Lack of self-esteem is often characterized by minimal mouth opening, reduced articulatory precision and vocal projection, and inappropriate resonance. Extreme tension in the mechanism, especially in the pharyngeal area, retracted tongue posture, and the substitution of laryngeal movements to compensate for inadequate velopharyngeal activity may be observed in adolescents with faulty learning, hearing impairment, or mild velopharyngeal inadequacy. "Deafy" voice is characterized by muffled (cul-de-sac) resonance, articulatory imprecision, and an inappropriate balance of nasal and oral resonance.

An appropriate balance of nasal and oral resonance may be affected by the degree of mouth opening and by lip and tongue movement. Any condition that constrains mouth and tongue movement (e.g., Bell's palsy, depression, orthodontic appliances, or glossitis) may be pertinent to the resonance characteristics of the voice.

♦ PSYCHOSOCIAL FACTORS

Voice is the most direct channel through which thoughts and feelings are shared. The way others react to the voice influences the way individuals think and feel about themselves. Human communication is dynamic and circular, and vocal behavior is an intrinsic and critical component of interpersonal interactions.

Sound self-esteem and satisfying interpersonal relationships correlate highly with vocal well-being. When vocal behavior causes difficulties, there is always some deleterious effect on self-concept and relationships (both intimate and casual). The degree of disruption will vary, but some disruption will always occur. That is why clinicians always need to address the social and emotional effects of any vocal disorder. No problem exists in a discrete form. Any problem that affects the ability to communicate creates social and emotional difficulties. Similarly, social and emotional problems can themselves create or exacerbate communication disorders. These interrelationships are what make differential diagnosis so challenging.

Sometimes, an individual's ego development, personality structure, and/or coping strategies give rise to atypical vocal behaviors. For example, voice symptoms may be indicative of internal distress, disorientation, or disintegration. Personality disorders can be the root cause of absent or distorted phonation, as can psycho-sexual conflicts. Thus, withdrawal of the self can be demonstrated through muteness, aphonia, or dysphonia. The lack of, or distortion of voice is then a symptom of the internal distress of the individual, and volitional control is absent or diminished.

Life stresses that an individual cannot confront directly are sometimes dealt with by using the voice as a defense to ward off pain or to protect and shield the ego. Conversion reactions are an extreme example of this, and in such instances the person is aphonic or severely dysphonic. Aronson (1980) defined a psychogenic voice disorder as the manifestation of one or more types of psychological disequilibrium where normal volitional control is suspended or disrupted.

The degree and type of interference with volitional control influences the number, type, and severity of the symptoms. There is a continuum of psychogenic disorders ranging from acute, short-term reactions to interpersonal conflicts or environmental stress, to chronically debilitating psychotic disorders.

Sometimes abuse and misuse of the voice, musculoskeletal states, and hyperfunction or hypofunction of muscle patterns result in structural changes in the vocal mechanism. What began as maladaptive behavior due to psychological disequilibrium develops into a problem with organic components. Conversely, an organically based problem may be compounded by psychosocial overlays. In some instances, precipitating and maintaining factors (e.g., secondary gains) interweave in complex patterns, and defense mechanisms, anxieties, learned behaviors, and compensations proliferate.

When vocal problems are part of a cluster of psychosocial difficulties, the speech-language pathologist may play a major role in helping adolescents learn more adult behaviors as a result of working through their difficulties. Vocal psychotherapy (Cooper, 1973) is frequently useful with adolescents. Adolescents often adopt roles or act inappropriately as a means of communication or as a way of testing whether adults can be trusted. They also experiment to test limits that are set by significant adults. Troubled adolescents may relate to a "neutral" adult (such as a speech-language pathologist) more easily and comfortably than to teachers or counselors. "Working on speech and voice" may seem less threatening and stigmatizing than seeking psychological counseling. A speech-language pathologist is often perceived as a professional who has no direct responsibility for grading academic performance. This can help students feel more open and less defensive. They may also feel more comfortable in revealing the general disequilibrium underlying their vocal symptoms. Speech-language pathologists are usually skilled communicators who can give support and direction and accept ambivalence and inconsistency with a certain amount of tolerance. Because their students are usually seen in individual or small group settings, they can relate to each student in a more personal way than a busy classroom teacher can. This individualized attention is what so many adolescents seem to crave. Thus, speech-language pathologists are sometimes in unique positions to intervene with adolescents who have adjustment difficulties related to self-concept and interpersonal relationships. Such students are frequently receptive to "trying out" new communication styles and testing and analyzing new strategies. Participation in situationally based activities is often seen as particularly "relevant" by adolescents. Mild-to-moderate psychosocial problems in combination with communication disorders can usually be dealt with most effectively by a skilled speech-language pathologist.

When a speech-language pathologist finds that a communication problem is related to a severe or global personality disorder (i.e., when the student is consistently unable to control behavior), more specialized assistance will be needed. Referrals for psychological or medical evaluation may be necessary, and a team approach to treatment may be needed. Even in cases of severe psychosocial dysfunction, the speech-language pathologist is usually part of the intervention team and collaborates closely with other professionals during the implementation of treatment programs.

APPENDIX TO CHAPTER 2
Conditions Affecting Vocal Tract Function

Altered Structures

1. Respiratory (subglottal)
   a. Anomalies
   b. Inflammatory conditions
   c. Sequela of trauma/surgical procedures
   d. Systemic diseases
   e. Neurological diseases
   f. Muscular/skeletal disorders
   g. Atypical secretions
2. Laryngeal (glottal)
   a. Anomalies (congenital/ maturational)
   b. Sequelae of trauma/surgical procedures
   c. Paresis/paralysis of folds
   d. Inflammatory conditions
   e. Vascular lesions
   f. Additive lesions of folds
   g. Chemically induced tissue change
   h. Hormonally induced tissue change
   i. Systemic diseases
   j. Gastroesophageal reflux
   k. Atypical secretions
3. Craniofacial (Supraglottal)
   a. Anomalies
   b. Sequelae of trauma/surgical procedures
   c. Paresis/paralysis of muscles
   d. Rhinological obstruction
   e. Temporomandibular joint (TMJ) dysfunction
   f. Inflammatory conditions
   g. Vascular lesions
   h. Systemic diseases
   i. Atypical secretions

Altered Sensory Feedback

   a. Hearing impairment
   b. Cerebral palsy
   c. Neurological deficits

   d. Orthodontic appliances
   e. Structural (temporary or permanent) constraints on vocal mechanism (tonsils/ adenoids)

Emotional/Psychosocial Conditions

   a. Atypical development
   b. Depression and other mental health dysfunctions
   c. Faulty learning/habits
   d. Conversion reactions
   e. Muscular tension/tics
   f. Psychosexual disorders

Musculoskeletal Conditions

   a. Diseases
   b. Cerebral palsy
   c. Hypertonic/hypotonic muscles
   d. Poor posture
   e. Compensatory behavioral patterns

Cognitive Conditions

   a. Mental retardation
   b. Learning disability
   c. Lack of awareness of cause/ effect relationships
   d. Poor motivation for self-improvement

Lifestyles Factors

   a. Time spent in vocally demanding activities
   b. Substance abuse
   c. Physical activities/mouth breathing
   d. Family's vocal style/models/ values
   e. Noise level in home
   f. Family history of vocal problems
   g. Sleep habits
   h. Nutrition

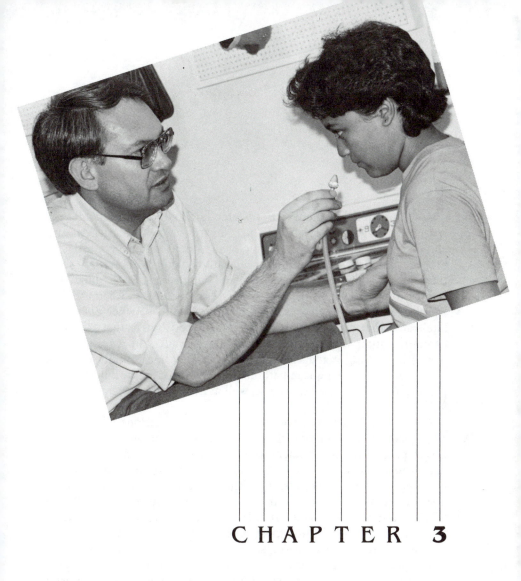

C H A P T E R **3**

Evaluation

Unfortunately, there are no standardized tests available for speech-language pathologists to use during voice diagnosis. In the absence of standardized tests, clinicians frequently develop a series of tasks designed to elicit samples of relevant behaviors. From these samples, the appropriateness of the voice is determined. Such subjective impressions are often difficult to record and classify systematically. Pannbacker (1984) reviewed classification systems of voice disorders. She stated that classifications need to be used in ways that facilitate communication with other professionals as well as in ways that are useful in making management decisions. This is especially true for the school speech-language pathologist, who must communicate with parents and other professionals, as well as be the major designer of the voice managment plan.

A speech-language pathologist faces other decisions when structuring the voice evaluation. These include selecting appropriate diagnostic procedures, an efficient system of recording and synthesizing data, and an effective way of translating diagnostic information into meaningful therapy objectives. Although excellent descriptions of assessment methods appear in texts such as Wilson (1979), Boone (1983), Aronson (1980), and Fox (1978), clinicians frequently want additional assistance in adapting these procedures for use with adolescents.

Speech-language pathologists need to collect and assimilate as much pertinent information as possible. The case conferencing procedure requires a succinct, yet thorough, presentation of diagnostic information. However, time constraints demand that a speech-language pathologist collect and summarize diagnostic information as efficiently as possible.

A convenient way to organize the vocal diagnostic process is to consider three general areas of behavior relevant to voice production: respiration, phonation, and resonance. However, it must be remembered that these three general areas are neither discrete nor all-inclusive. A student's behavior during diagnostic sessions provides only part of the information necessary to determine appropriate referrals and management strategies. A student's problem must be seen in a wider context, and information from additional sources must be integrated with data on respiration, phonation, and resonance.

Certain physical, psychological, and sociological factors, individually or in combination, can heighten susceptibility to the development and maintenance of a vocal disorder. For example, conditions of the upper respiratory tract, such as chronic infections or allergic reactions, may place a vocally active student, such as a cheerleader, at greater risk than a student with a less vocally demanding lifestyle. High risk factors relating specifically to the adolescent lifestyle must be identified and considered.

A speech-language pathologist needs to observe a student and gain supplementary information from school personnel concerning the student's patterns of interaction, coping strategies, and favored activities. During the vocally active middle and high school years, students engage in many activities (e.g., cheerleading, athletics, debate, dramatic productions, choral activities, lengthy telephone conversations) that place unusual demands on the vocal mechanism. The transition from childhood to adulthood results in physiological changes of the mechanism and psychological stress. In an effort to cope with stressful situations, some students engage in crying jags, alcohol and drug abuse, and loud attention-getting behaviors. There is some evidence that eating disorders, such as anorexia nervosa (which lowers the body's resistance to infection) and bulimia (with frequent spasmodic contractions of the trachea and esophagus combined with acidic secretions) may heighten the risk of vocal problems.

Evaluating vocal risk is often challenging because there are so many pertinent risk factors to be considered in relation to a student's medical history, family situation, lifestyle demands, and interpersonal relationships. The most important aspects of this task are (1) considering all relevant risk factors, (2) condensing information into a manageable format, and (3) integrating information concerning the relationship of risk factors to each other and to data collected from traditional areas of evaluation (respiration, phonation, and resonance). When this is accomplished successfully, the collected information results in a comprehensive picture of a student's voice problem presented in a manageable format. The speech-language pathologist can then easily retrieve pertinent information and identify appropriate management strategies.

The organizational system outlined in this chapter is presented so that therapy planning arises naturally from collected data. The evaluation form contains traditional questions on respiration, phonation, and resonance, as well as sample tasks designed to target critical behaviors that are prerequisites for appropriate vocal production (Figures 3-1 through 3-3). The evaluation also covers high-risk factors: physical conditions, abusive practices, demands inherent in lifestyle and environment, and interpersonal behaviors (Figure 3-4). A "skipping option" is provided in each section to shorten the in-depth evaluation for students who demonstrate appropriate behavior in certain areas of performance. For example, a student who demonstrates appropriate behaviors in a general area, such as resonance, need only be checked as "appropriate." Demographic information, a summary of areas to be considered in therapy, recommendations, and referrals should also be recorded. This facilitates the easy retrieval of pertinent information for case conferences and therapy planning.

◆ RESPIRATION

If there are indications that respiration may be inappropriate for speech, the speech-language pathologist completes six items designed to record characteristics of a student's breathing pattern (Figure 3-1). Information for items A and B may be obtained by observing a student

FIGURE 3-1.
Evaluation Form: Respiration

Respiration for speech appears appropriate _____ inappropriate _____.
A. Inspiration: appropriate _____ shallow _____ audible breathing _____
B. Tension sites: none _____ upper chest _____ neck _____
C. Length of exhalation
   1. Counts on one breath to _____ (note number)
   2. Sustains s-s-s _____ secs.
   3. Sustains z-z-z _____ secs.
   4. Sustains /a/ _____ secs.
   Ratio of s/z = _____*
   Average maximum phonation time: _____
D. Control of exhalation (stopping and starting airflow)
   Number of /h/ productions per exhalation:
   trial 1 _____ trial 2 _____ trial 3 _____
E. Use of replenishing breaths
   1. number of breaths taken while counting to 50 _____
   2. number of breaths taken while reading (50 words at reading level) _____
F. Coordination of respiration with phonatory demands in spontaneous speech is
   rhythmical _____ arrhythmical _____ .

*Is the s/z ratio noted above greater than or equal to 1.20:1? yes _____ no _____. If yes, the possibility of laryngeal pathology exists and medical referral should be made.

during a spontaneous speech sample involving connected speech for approximately two minutes.

Since voicing occurs during the exhalation phase of speech breathing, it is helpful to determine the length of the exhalation and maximum phonation time (item C). Typically, prepubertal children prolong consonants (Tait, Michel, & Carpenter, 1980) and vowels (Wilson (1979) of approximately 10 seconds' duration. In the adolescent age range, 10 seconds should be regarded as a minimal proficiency level. Higher levels (i.e., adults levels of 20 to 25 seconds) would be necessary for students with vocally demanding lifestyles (Ptacek & Sander, 1963).

It is critical to observe the relationship between the prolongation of /s/ and /z/ (Eckel & Boone, 1981). A student who prolongs the unvoiced /s/ for a significantly longer time than the voiced /z/, obviously has adequate available air supply and can sustain flow, but is experiencing difficulty at the laryngeal valving level. A student who demonstates an s/z ratio of 2:1 should be referred for laryngeal examination. Prater and Swift (1984) recommended that a cutoff ratio of 1.20:1 be used to determine the need for laryngeal evaluation. This means that a student who, on repeated trials, sustains /s/ for 18 seconds and /z/ for 15 seconds should be referred for medical evaluation, even though the length of the exhalation falls within normal limits.

After a student has been given clear instructions, a model, and practice trials, an averaged performance on prolongation of /a/ that falls below 10 seconds could suggest inadequate respiration, inadequate laryngeal valving (laryngeal pathology, such as nodules), neurologic involvement, or faulty learning of the coordination of air flow with voicing.

Since running speech involves segmentation of air flow during the exhalation phase, it is helpful to observe a student's ability to interrupt the continuity of airflow. The task in item D (Figure 3-1) involves the production of the unvoiced phoneme /h/. This is to ensure that respiratory activity can be observed in the absence of laryngeal valving or articulatory interruption of airflow. Space for three trials is provided to ensure that a student is comfortable with the task and is given an opportunity to improve performance with practice. Instructions and a model should be provided.

To produce smooth, connected utterances, a student must be able to use replenishing breaths in ways that do not detract from the content of a message (items E and F, Figure 3-1). Therefore, the frequency, obtrusiveness, and timing of these breaths must be observed in both automatic and spontaneous speech samples, as well as in a predetermined linguistic pattern (e.g., reading a passage). The advantage of including a predetermined linguistic pattern is that it can also be used as a post-test later in the therapy program.

◆ **PHONATION**

If phonatory behavior appears inappropriate in quality, onset, loudness, pitch, or rate, the speech-language pathologist should evaluate the inappropriate dimensions (Figure 3-2). However, it is usually advantageous to evaluate all dimensions of phonation to obtain comprehensive information.

To observe the quality of a student's voice, the speech-language pathologist should elicit prolongations and then a spontaneous speech sample of at least 2 minutes in duration. It is important to have the student prolong the consonants /s/ and /z/, since the s/z ratio provides information concerning vocal fold pathology (Eckel & Boone, 1981). The prolongation of /a/ provides an opportunity to evaluate characteristics such as pitch breaks, aphonic episodes, and diplophonia. A reading passage is also useful since some people adopt a different phonatory style during reading. Since students with vocal nodules frequently produce a clearer voice quality during higher-pitched or louder speech, this can be observed by asking the student to recite the months of the year, first in a higher voice, then in a louder voice. Since hormonal fluctuations during the menstrual cycle may result in swelling of the laryngeal and/or nasal mucosa, female students should be questioned to ascertain possible changes in voice quality prior to and during menstruation.

The appropriate timing and coordination of air flow with the onset of phonation (item C) is a prerequisite for effective vocal production. When the relationship between air flow and onset is disturbed, the appropriate initiation of phonation should become a therapy goal.

A vocally abusive practice frequently seen in students with voice disorders is the hard glottal attack. Items C1-C7 provide opportunities to observe the type of onset during the production of stressed syllables beginning with vowels, since this is the context in which hard attacks are most likely to occur. Examples of sentences to be repeated in a loud voice are included in the evaluation form to identify the frequency of occurrence of hard attacks in relation to loudness level (items 8-11, Figure 3-2). Finally, the type of onset most frequently occurring during spontaneous speech should be noted.

Many people with voice disorders, especially those whose disorders are related to vocal abuse, may habituate excessively loud vocal behavior and limited control and variability of loudness patterns (item

FIGURE 3-2.

Evaluation Form: Phonation

Rate the following dimensions of phonatory behavior:

	quality	onset	loudness	pitch	rate
appropriate	_____	_____	_____	_____	_____
inappropriate	_____	_____	_____	_____	_____

A. Quality in sustained phonation
   1. Sustains s-s-s _____ secs. ⎫
   2. Sustains z-z-z _____ secs. ⎬ Ratio of s/z = _____*
   3. Sustains /a/ _____ secs. ⎭

   Average maximum phonation time _____ .

B. Quality in spontaneous speech sample
   1. Breathy _____ mild _____ moderate _____ severe _____
   2. Harsh _____ mild _____ moderate _____ severe _____
   3. Hoarse _____ mild _____ moderate _____ severe _____
   4. Related observations: pitch breaks _____ phonation breaks _____
      aphonia _____ glottal fry _____ diplophonia _____ tremor _____
      other _____
   5. How does a higher pitch affect quality? improves _____ worsens _____
      no change _____
   6. How does a louder level affect quality? improves _____ worsens _____
      no change _____
   7. Is quality affected by menstrual cycle? yes _____ no _____

C. Onset of phonation

In single words	appropriate	breathy	hard glottal
1. arm /a/	_____	_____	_____
2. eggs /e/	_____	_____	_____
3. umpire /ʌ/	_____	_____	_____
4. out /au/	_____	_____	_____
5. ooze /u/	_____	_____	_____
6. eight /eI/	_____	_____	_____
7. apple /æ/	_____	_____	_____

   In sentences (to be said loudly)

	appropriate	breathy	hard glottal
8. Allen Edwards is engaged to Erica Underwood.	_____	_____	_____
9. Is everyone awfully angry?	_____	_____	_____
10. Amy Anderson always understands.	_____	_____	_____
11. Extra actors are out at the entrance.	_____	_____	_____

   In spontaneous speech
   (conversational level) _____ _____ _____

D. Loudness
   1. Prolonged vowel loudly _____ sec.
   2. Prolonged vowel softly _____ sec.
   3. Sustained vowels gradually increasing and decreasing loudness
      Ability to control loudness: yes _____ no _____

(continued)

FIGURE 3-2. *(continued)*

Limited loudness range: yes _____ no _____
Tension present: yes _____ no _____ when _____

4. Counting from soft to loud, loud to soft
   Ability to control variation: yes _____ no _____
   Limited range: yes _____ no _____
   Tension present: yes _____ no _____ when _____

5. Level during reading passage: overstrong _____ weak _____
   fading _____ lacking in variety _____ inappropriate to meaning _____
   tension present_____

6. Level during spontaneous speech: overstrong _____ weak _____
   fading _____ lacking in variety _____ inappropriate to meaning _____
   tension present_____

E. Pitch observed during reading _____ spontaneous speech _____ both _____
   1. Habitual level
      a. Appropriate to age and sex _____ too low _____ too high_____
      b. Does the student's age and physical development indicate the possibility of
         pubertal voice changes? yes _____ no _____
   2. Voice breaks to higher pitch _____ lower pitch _____
   3. Variability
      a. Amount: appropriate _____ limited _____ monotone _____
         exaggerated _____
      b. Consistency of use of pitch changes to reflect meaning:
         always _____ sometimes _____ never _____
   4. Ability to produce extremes of pitch range (isolated vowels):
      good _____ fair _____ poor_____
   5. Ability to discriminate pitch differences (isolated tones, series of tones):
      good _____ fair _____ poor_____
   6. Ability to imitate a given pitch (isolated vowels):
      good _____ fair _____ poor_____
   7. Ability to imitate sequential pitch patterns (series of vowels):
      good _____ fair _____ poor_____
   8. Ability to imitate pitch inflections (phrases, e.g., It's mine? vs. It's mine!):
      good _____ fair _____ poor_____

F. Rate (in spontaneous speech):
   too fast _____ too slow _____ arrhythmical _____

G. Phrasing errors
   insufficient replenishing breaths _____   lack of smoothness _____
   inappropriate to meaning _____   inappropriate pause lengths ____
   limited variety _____   dysfluencies _____

* Is the s/z ratio noted above greater than or equal to 1.20:1? yes _____ no _____ If yes,
the possibility of laryngeal pathology exists and medical referral should be made.

D). The ability to produce a clear phonation at a soft level is often difficult for the student with vocal pathology. The presence or absence of observable tension can indicate the relationship between effort and output. The pattern of habitual loudness level may also be significant. For example, if a student's voice consistently fades at the end of sentences, it may suggest a relationship between available air supply and loudness.

Precise adjustments of the laryngeal musculature in association with control of air flow are necessary to produce appropriate pitch patterns. Conditions of the vocal folds, such as edema, inflammation, growths, or neurological deficits, interfere with these adjustments. Since nodules are a frequently occurring vocal pathology, it is important to note that the resulting changes in the mass of the folds may be reflected in inappropriate pitch behavior.

It is important to note the influence age or physical maturity may exert on vocal characteristics and to note the direction of voice breaks, since clinical observation suggests that a voice breaks in the direction it wishes to go (Figure 3-2). Variability of the voice may be affected by such factors as environmental models, neurological or cognitive deficits, emotional state, and hearing acuity. If a student's variability of pitch is limited, items 4 and 5 (Figure 3-2) can be used to assess available pitch range and pitch discrimination ability. When a student is able to imitate both isolated and sequenced pitches, but does not employ meaningful variation spontaneously, the use of pitch changes to reflect thoughts and feelings could be an appropriate therapy goal. However, lack of vocal variation in adolescents may indicate depression. A student's general demeanor and facial expression are further indicators of emotional state.

◆ RESONANCE

An appropriate resonance pattern is the result of a balance of direct nasal resonance (on /m/, /n/, and /ŋ/), indirect nasal resonance, and oral resonance (all vowels and non-nasal consonants). Hypernasality, or an excess of direct nasal resonance on sounds other than /m/, /n/, and /ŋ/, may indicate velopharyngeal inadequacy, whereas hyponasality, or an absence of direct nasal resonance on /m/, /n/, and /ŋ/, may indicate acute or chronic nasal congestion or other obstruction. It is important to emphasize the need for medical referral if hyponasality or hypernasality is noted. Although inappropriate resonance may be the result of faulty learning, the presence of organic impairment must always be carefully explored before attempting behavioral modification. Fluctuations in resonance patterns may also indicate the early onset of neurological disease or, in girls, intermittent swelling of the nasal mucosa related to menstrual cycles.

If resonance appears inappropriate for speech, the speech-language pathologist completes eight items designed to record a student's resonance characteristics (Figure 3-3). Items A, B, and C (Figure 3-3) allow the speech-language pathologist to explore the possibility of hyponasality. It may be valuable to occlude the nares one at a time while the student is humming to determine the presence of a nostril obstruction (item A). Occluding the nares in item B can help the speech-language pathologist determine if an obstruction is total or partial. In the absence of an obstruction, direct nasal resonance will be normal when the nares are not occluded. Characteristics that are indicative of adenoidal enlargement, tissue changes in the nasal cavity, or upper respiratory conditions should be noted in item C.

Items D, E, and F (Figure 3-3) allow the speech-language pathologist to explore the possibility of hypernasalsity. Inadequate velopharyngeal closure may be indicated if the sentences in item E sound more appropriate when spoken with both nares occluded than with both nares open. Characteristics frequently associated with velopharyngeal inadequacy are listed in item F. The Iowa Pressure Test, a subtest of the Templin-Darley (Morris, Spriesterbach, & Darley, 1961) may be used to explore further the articulation of pressure consonants.

Items G and H (Figure 3-3) focus on the ability to valve appropriately on sequences of oral and nasal sounds. Contrasting word pairs allow the clinician to observe changes related to the effect of nasal consonants on vowels. The conversation and reading sample can show the overall effect of the resonance pattern in connected speech. The influence of associated articulatory behaviors on resonance during conversational and projected speech should be noted in item J.

◆ HIGH-RISK FACTORS

It is clear that certain physical and emotional factors, as well as learned or habituated behaviors, may (1) increase susceptibility to developing a voice disorder (e.g., upper respiratory conditions), (2) maintain or reinforce inappropriate vocal use (e.g., cheerleading, throat clearing), (3) provide secondary gains for an individual (e.g., attention-getting behaviors such as impersonations), or (4) result in compensatory behaviors that compound the original problem (e.g., hyperextended jaw, coughing). Noting the risk factors during an evaluation (Figure 3-4) helps a speech-language pathologist to determine the need for referral to other professionals and to determine the

FIGURE 3-3.

Evaluation Form: Resonance

Overall resonance in reading and conversation:
appropriate _____ inappropriate _____

A. Nasal resonance while sustaining a hum:
weak _____ absent _____ appropriate _____

B. Nasal sentences (to check for hyponasality)
Mary Morgan makes me mad. (nares open)
Mary Morgan makes me mad. (nares occluded) } same _____ different _____
Neal knows Nathan's never neat. (nares open)
Neal knows Nathan's never neat. (nares occluded) } same _____ different _____

C. Observed characteristics of nasal obstruction:
swelling/dark circles under eyes _____ noisy breathing _____ mouth breathing _____
swelling of nasal bridge _____ discharge _____ congestion _____
enlarged tonsils _____ snoring _____ deviated septum _____
Comments: _____

D. Prolonged /a/: nasal emission is absent _____ present _____

E. Oral sentences (to check for hypernasality)
She eats sweet peas. (nares open)
She eats sweet peas (nares occluded) } same _____ different _____
Charley chews potato chips. (nares open)
Charley chews potato chips. (nares occluded) } same _____ different _____

F. Observed characteristics of velopharyngeal inadequacy:
snorts _____ grimaces _____ nares constriction _____ nasal emission _____
palatal deviations _____ distortion of pressure consonants _____
Comments: _____

G. Word pairs (vowels in non-nasal vs. nasal contexts):

	appropriate	hypernasal	hyponasal	assimil. nasality on vowels only
hat/ham	_____	_____	_____	_____
pat/mat	_____	_____	_____	_____
bat/man	_____	_____	_____	_____
towel/town	_____	_____	_____	_____
how/now	_____	_____	_____	_____
pout/noun	_____	_____	_____	_____

H. Oral–nasal balance (during conversation and/or reading):
appropriate _____ hypernasal _____ hyponasal _____ mixed _____
cul-de-sac (muffled) _____

I. Tone focus (when counting):

	seated near clinician		projecting voice across room	
	adequate	inadequate	adequate	inadequate
mouth opening	_____	_____	_____	_____
lip movement	_____	_____	_____	_____
tongue movement (retracted?)	_____	_____	_____	_____
supraglottal tension	_____	_____	_____	_____

FIGURE 3-4.
Evaluation Form: High-Risk Factors

High-risk factors appear to be present _____ absent _____.
A. **Physical conditions** that may be pertinent:
hearing loss _____ craniofacial anomalies _____ hyperextended jaw _____
allergies _____ deviated septum _____ surgery _____ abnormal palate _____
frequent upper respiratory infections _____ medications _____
asymetrical/weak palatal movement on /a →ŋ/ _____ postnasal drip _____
bifid uvula _____ neurological symptoms _____ excessive mucus _____
hormonal problem _____ cerebral palsy _____ mouth breathing _____
mental retardation _____ enlarged tonsils/adenoids _____
atypical tongue carriage _____ learning disability _____ anorexia nervosa _____
premenstrual syndrome _____ dentition/orthodontia _____
Other: _____
Comments: _____
B. **Abusive practices:**
throat clearing _____ crying _____ excessive talking _____
strained laughing _____ screaming _____ impersonations _____
coughing _____ smoking _____ competing with background noise _____
yodeling _____ grunting _____ bulimia _____
sings along with records/tapes/radio _____ cheering _____
Other: _____
Comments: _____
C. **Factors inherent in lifestyle/environment:**
voice models _____ noisy environment _____ cheerleading _____ sports _____
choir/singing _____ poor sleep/poor eating habits _____ dramatics _____
debate _____ stress _____ family communication style _____ air pollution _____
Other: _____
Comments: _____
D. **Interpersonal behaviors:**
talking too much _____ ignoring feedback _____ not seeking feedback _____
ignoring differences between people _____ ignoring differences in situations _____
ignoring needs and interests of others _____ poor self-esteem _____
depression _____ aggressive behavior _____ competing for attention _____
emotional lability _____
Other: _____
Comments: _____

influence risk factors have on the therapy prognosis. Recognizing risk factors facilitates the design of a voice therapy program that is relevant to a student, that incorporates factors in the student's physical environment that should be modified (e.g., TV/stereo level at home), and that isolates factors that can be addressed through consultation with parents and teachers.

Item D (Figure 3-4) focuses attention on the important area of interpersonal behavior. Self-esteem and relations with others affect vocal effectiveness. Although research does not indicate that students with voice disorders also exhibit interpersonal problems, clinical experience suggests that voice problems may be exacerbated by poor interpersonal skills. It is often necessary for speech-language pathologists to incorporate therapy goals designed to restructure patterns of interpersonal interaction. For example, a student who talks incessantly in a loud voice may be unaware of the effect this behavior has on others and may need to learn to observe others' reactions to communicate more effectively. In addition, the student may need to learn that getting louder is not the most effective way to hold a listener's attention. A therapy goal for such a person might be to use various vocal options (pitch, rate, inflection) to increase communication effectivenes.

Since most public school speech-language pathologists do not have access to sophisticated laboratory equipment, this evaluation system does not require the use of any instrumentation. However, additional information obtained by the use of portable equipment (e.g., Visipitch by Kay Elemetrics) can easily be added to the evaluation form.

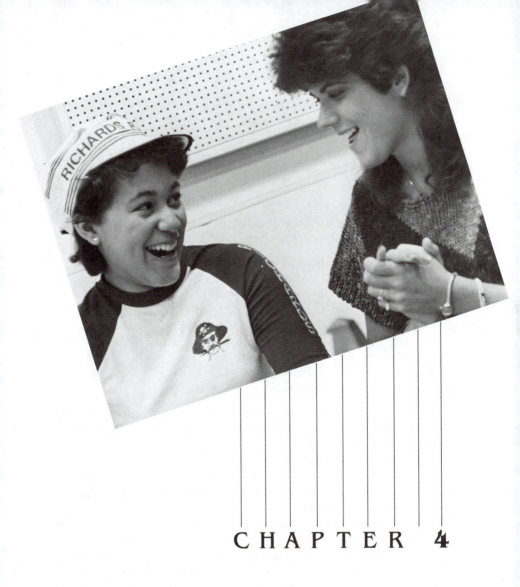

CHAPTER 4

Establishing a
Therapeutic Partnership

V oice therapy is a process that begins with the initial meeting and covers a series of stages including:

♦ growth of the therapeutic relationship
♦ exploration of the client's concerns and vocal symptoms
♦ determination of goals
♦ development of an individualized approach to achieving goals (contract negotiation, when appropriate)
♦ implementation of an individualized approach to achieving goals
♦ evaluation of results
♦ termination and follow-up.

Prior to their initial contact, the speech-language pathologist and the student are usually strangers. They bring vastly different orientations, perspectives, and expectations to their first meeting. Each may have heard about the other by reputation, but neither is likely to know much about the other as an individual. For success to be achieved, they must learn to interact as partners. The quality of the therapeutic partnership is of great significance. It undergirds the predictable stages of the intervention process and is crucial to its outcome. That is not to say that students and clinicians must become close friends. There is a difference between a professional partnership and a personal relationship, and it is usually counterproductive for an adult to try to interact with an adolescent as if they were peers.

It is imperative that a speech-language pathologist be concerned with the adolescent as an individual — that is, as a person rather than as a person with a voice defect. If the speech-language pathologist allows sufficient time at the outset of the intervention process to learn about the student as a whole person (rather than as just a set of disordered symptoms), a useful framework for the intervention program will evolve.

Before a speech-language pathologist and student can develop a shared sense of their mission, they must have a clear definition of their roles. Many students approach voice therapy believing that the speech-language pathologist will "fix" their voice. They may not understand the interactive nature of the therapy process. Speech-language pathologists, on the other hand, may believe that a student should enter the relationship with an understanding of the problem, a commitment to change, and an unconditional trust in the therapist's expertise.

It is important to remember that adolescents enter voice therapy at different levels of readiness. Many students "test" speech-language pathologists to be sure that they can be trusted and have the ability to help. Some students approach voice therapy hoping to hold the speech-language pathologist responsible for its outcome. Students who have been pressured to seek help may be uncomfortable, defensive, or hostile. Their hostility can be expressed openly (as in the case of defiant behavior) or in more subtle ways. Some of the passive ways in which hostility may be expressed are digressions, reticence, substituting another issue for the real issue, pretending to cooperate, joking or avoiding the real issue, and minimizing the problem.

All speech-language pathologists should be sensitive to the inevitable differences between their own and the student's views of roles and expectations in the voice therapy process. A major task in voice therapy is to mesh perceptions and expectations to build a workable partnership.

Equality in an interaction is communicated in many ways, both verbal and nonverbal. Speaking and listening time should be roughly equal, and disagreements should be seen as predictable means of solving problems rather than as power plays. Equality does not mean never challenging another's behavior, but it does mean accepting another's rights. Equal relationships are generally supportive relationships, since no one is attempting to win or prove superiority. The way questions are asked is often an indication of the way one person feels about another. Questions asked in a demanding way presume compliance and frequently result in defensive or resentful responses. Consider, for example, how "Have you forgotten to do your assignment again? Why don't you write it down next time?" communicates superiority. The clinician is not presenting a cooperative approach to problem solving, and the questions reflect it.

If a student has had previous experience in a speech or voice therapy program, an exploration of reactions and feelings to what occurred is in order. If the speech-language pathologist is accepting of the student's negative, as well as positive, reactions, this information-sharing can enhance their relationship and provide valuable insights for future programming.

A speech-language pathologist may find students reluctant to share information for numerous reasons. Students will feel inhibited if information they divulge can be used against them or if they are criticized or made to feel foolish. Many students are reluctant to divulge information that violates the privacy of events occurring within the family. Adolescents often find it difficult to express painful feelings and may try to repress feelings such as guilt, embarrassment, and anger because these feelings seem less painful if ignored. Feelings that diminish an individual's sense of adequacy are especially threatening to the self-concept. For example, an adolescent male may be reluctant to report information about situations in which his voice was perceived as "unmanly." Divulging such information could come in conflict with the emerging masculinity he is trying so hard to project.

The clinician must listen to the literal meaning of a student's communication and be sensitive to other levels of meaning. Nonverbal communication may provide critical information concerning the student and, frequently, the style of communication is significant. For example, the student who continually challenges content may not merely be debating the issues. Such a student may be signalling objections to the clinician's authoritarian approach. On the other hand, such a student may have a more general problem in relating to adults. Indeed, some teenagers seem to go from the submissiveness of childhood to an aggressive "question authority" mode of operation without ever exploring the value and pleasure of a cooperative, interactive style.

The active listener considers both verbal and nonverbal signals and is sensitive to the underlying as well as literal meanings of messages. When students express disappointments, the sensitive listener responds in ways that accept the validity of their feelings. When a listener uses strategies that acknowledge negative feelings, more open communication follows.

When barriers, such as defensiveness or an unwillingness to trust the clinician, interfere with the growth of the therapeutic relationship, the clinician may adopt an indirect approach. Some clinicians prefer not to "press" too hard, fearing that a defensive client will become more intimidated and less open. If a clinician feels that a student's sense-of-self is particularly fragile, an indirect approach, in which the student's unwillingness to share information is not challenged, may be adopted. The clinician may observe the student's indirect refusal to deal with the central problem in behaviors such as evasion of significant issues during discussion, emphasis on peripheral information, or denial of negative feelings. A student who repeatedly states that others are overreacting to the voice problem or who denies concern about a voice problem is exhibiting a lack of readiness to deal with the central problem.

In an indirect approach, the speech-language pathologist focuses attention on general information and allows students to internalize at their own pace. In the direct approach, the speech-language pathologist challenges students in a supportive, nonthreatening manner, to apply specific insights to their own particular situations. For example, "During our discussions I have noticed that you have been saying very little. I know it might be difficult for you, but it would help me to understand how you really feel if you could give me some examples of times when you feel your voice has let you down."

A speech-language pathologist must always be concerned with the development of a trusting relationship when working with the adolescent. A student needs to feel free to talk about personal concerns and feelings in a nonthreatening environment and must be aware that confidences will not be betrayed. Rogers (1961) and Truax and Carkhuff (1967) stated that empathy, genuineness, and positive regard on the part of a counselor helps to facilitate a sense of trust and open communication.

♦ ENCOURAGING SELF-DISCLOSURE AND PARTICIPATION

Self-disclosure helps adolescents gain a new sense of themselves and a deeper understanding of their own behavior. Self-acceptance is difficult without self-disclosure. Frequently, it is not the clinician who identifies salient issues, but students who see new aspects of their behavior. The following guidelines can help a speech-language pathologist encourage self-disclosure:

♦ Be an effective and active listener (give verbal and nonverbal responses).
♦ Listen for different levels of meaning.
♦ Listen with empathy.
♦ Listen with an open mind.
♦ Paraphrase the student to check understanding.
♦ Express understanding of the student's feelings.
♦ Ask questions to check understanding and to indicate interest.
♦ Provide support for the student. (Refrain from evaluations during disclosures, allow the student to set the pace, and signal support through verbal and nonverbal responses.)
♦ Maintain a climate of trust. (Keep information confidential, reinforce self-disclosing behaviors, show positive attitudes toward the student and the disclosures, maintain appropriate eye contact, don't use disclosed information against a student at a later date.)

♦ Avoid burdensome reciprocal disclosure. (Lengthy anecdotes from the speech-language pathologist may shift the focus away from the student.)

When a student begins the process of sharing personal information, it is important for the clinician to respond in ways that facilitate the continuation of productive dialogue. Some of the techniques frequently used to achieve this goal include:

♦ Paraphrasing (e.g., "You said you were nervous before speaking to the teacher.")
♦ Reflecting statements (e.g., "It seems that you are angry that she wanted you to come to voice therapy.")
♦ Clarifying information (e.g., "Could you tell me more about what you were doing when you lost your voice?")
♦ Clarifying feelings (e.g., "How do you feel when you anticipate giving a report before the class?")
♦ Making tentative inferences (e.g., "I have a hunch that it was a very difficult situation for you.")
♦ Sending "I" messages (e.g., "I am confused. Could you explain it once more?" the clinician assumes responsibility for not understanding).
♦ Affirming (e.g., You're giving me a good picture of the situation").

Empathetic probes can clarify the feelings associated with a student's description of events and circumstances. These statements are especially useful when a clinician senses a disparity between what a student is saying and how the student may actually have been feeling. The use of empathetic probes can provide support for what the student has said as well as further clarify what actual feelings were projected. Such probes should be used cautiously early in therapy, before trust and open communication have been fully developed. It can be intimidating to a student if a clinician seems to be inferring and interpreting too much too soon.

Carkhuff (1969) talked about additive empathy responses of this kind. He defines them as responses that "add significantly to the feeling and meaning of the expressions of the client ... The counselor responds with accuracy to all of the client's deeper as well as surface feelings" (p. 175). He contrasted these additive empathy responses with interchangeable empathy responses. Interchangeable empathy responses merely capture and reflect back to the client the essential part of the message. We have called Carkhuff's additive empathy responses "empathy probes" because they probe beyond the student's stated message.

Carkhuff (1969) stated that counseling is effective when a client experiences a developmental process of exploration leading to awareness, which leads to new actions. In voice therapy, as a student begins to explore feelings and underlying assumptions, an open relationship with the clinician allows for clarification of vague or confusing issues, the application of different ideas and information, and increased understanding of the motivations for behavior. Through continued examination, the student develops new insights and can decide how to practice new vocal behaviors in a variety of contexts.

The intervention process should proceed to a discussion of specific vocal behaviors only after a speech-language pathologist has become familiar with a student's interests, needs, social interaction, communication style, and aspirations. The clinician projects that the student is interesting as a person by not rushing in and pinpointing problems before understanding the student as a whole. In other words, the intervention process begins with due consideration of the person — not the problem. This assures the student that the clincian has adequate information and does not jump to conclusions or make suggestions without understanding the whole situation.

Too often, an experienced clinician concerned with the most efficient use of time feels compelled to "zero in" on vocal problems, describe them succinctly to the student, and prescribe appropriate strategies for behavior modification. This approach, although time-saving, may result in costly long-term consequences. Motivation is rarely encouraged by a clinician telling an adolescent what is wrong and what needs to be done to fix it. An adolescent's self-esteem is not enhanced by adult authority figures presenting ready-made solutions to problems. Rather than applauding the skill of the clinician who diagnoses a voice problem in 10 minutes, an adolescent may react with resentment, feeling that the clinician could not possibly understand the problem in so brief a time. The student may feel threatened and may resist the therapy plan to assert autonomy.

It is difficult for adolescents to become part of something as anxiety provoking as behavioral change. They first need to feel that they are accepted and understood as unique human beings and that they are involved in the change process. Anyone affected by change must "buy into" or "invest" in the project before change can truly be accepted. Rosabeth Kantner (1983), in her book *The Change Masters,* called this stage "tin cupping" — that is, giving those most affected by change the opportunity to throw "their two-cents worth" into the cup. The speech-language pathologist gives students this opportunity by allowing them adequate time to describe themselves, their aspirations, and their priorities. Feelings of self-worth are enhanced as students perceive that a clinician values the information they have to offer. Their shared insights can become intrinsic parts of a cooperative approach to problem-solving.

Adolescents are frequently difficult to motivate in situations in which they feel adults are forcing change on them. They frequently feel ambivalent about authority figures and may resent being singled out for specialized help. An adolescent may react against a parent or teacher's suggestion that voice therapy will be helpful. Since many teenagers need feelings of independence, extrinsic factors such as parental involvement in a therapy program may detract from the therapy outcome.

Involving students in the decision-making process assures them that a clinician has confidence in their abilities to control and chart their own futures. If some initial success can be achieved, it provides evidence that therapy is, indeed, worthwhile and creates additional momentum and enthusiasm.

♦ **WRITING A CONTRACT**

Since voice therapy with adolescents assumes a level of independence and self-determination on the part of the student, explicit contracts are methods for formalizing mutually agreed-on goals and expectations. Contracts can take various forms as long as they are mutually determined and not forced on a student. It is generally not a good idea to present a preplanned contractual agreement to a student. That is not to say an agreement should not be written, but rather the written format should evolve as a result of interaction between a speech-language pathologist and a student. Negotiations concerning the agreement are then an integral part of the learning process.

It is sometimes helpful, particularly with reticent students, for both the clinician and student to complete a set of open-ended questions independently, and then discuss these documents together. At other times, it may be helpful for the student to answer selected questions to increase the clinician's understanding of the student's perspective, expectations, and commitment (Figure 4–1).

Typically, a contract includes not only long-term objectives but also such requirements as attendance, division of responsibility, frequency of contacts with clinician, and termination criteria. A contract should also include dates for progress reviews and for termination, extension, or revision of the treatment plan, and a list of those who will receive copies of progress reports. It is helpful to add statements concerning the voice therapy approach and format. This is done to

FIGURE 4-1.

Student Questionaire

1. My purpose in therapy is _____ .
2. I am prepared to commit the following amount of time each day: _____
   _____ .
3. I am prepared to commit the following amount of time each week: _____
   _____ .
4. I expect this program to last approximately _____ .
5. I will discontinue therapy when _____ .
6. For my therapy, I feel that being grouped with other students
   _____ is desirable
   _____ is undesirable
   _____ is desirable on a limited basis
7. For my therapy, I feel that working individually with the pathologist is desirable
   _____ on a regular basis
   _____ on a limited basis
8. Where homework is concerned I feel that _____ .
9. The home assignment(s) I would most enjoy is/are _____ .
10. One type of home assignment I do not enjoy is _____ .
11. My parents' attitude to my problem is _____ .
12. My family should be involved in the following way _____ .
13. Significant others in my life view my problem as _____ .
14. My reaction to their help with my therapy program would be _____ .
15. When someone makes a recommendation to me I prefer that _____
    _____ .
16. I respond best to criticism when _____ .
17. Generally, I absorb new ideas best when _____ .
18. When I read a self-help book I am most likely to pay attention to _____
    _____
    _____ .
19. When I am tested I prefer _____ .
20. To solve problems I am likely to _____ .
21. I prefer therapy to be _____% with the pathologist, _____% with a group of
    other students, and _____% on my own.
22. When it comes to identifying errors, I prefer to
    _____ check myself.
    _____ have other students help check me.
    _____ have the speech-language pathologist check me.
    _____ have significant others check me.
23. In acquiring new information, I prefer to
    _____ have the speech-language pathologist verbally give me the information.
    _____ have the speech-language pathologist give me articles, etc.
    _____ go to the library and find the information I feel is relevant.

(continued)

FIGURE 4-1. *(continued)*

24. When I approach a problem I
_____ look for ways to get the problem solved quickly.
_____ think of a number of different ways to solve the problem.
_____ ask others for solutions.
_____ work out a step-by-step plan for solving the problem.
25. In making recommendations to me about my voice, I would prefer that the speech-language pathologist
_____ show how the recommendations would support my overall goals.
_____ outline a plan to implement the recommendations.
_____ tell me the drawbacks as well as the benefits of the recommendations.

maximize a student's investment in the program and to exploit the student's self-knowledge about preferred learning style.

In some middle and high school settings, the contract has been incorporated into the language arts curriculum so that a student in a speech-language pathology program can earn credit toward the language arts requirement. In such cases, requirements for a grade must be stipulated in the contract. Some speech-language pathologists offer an independent studies option in which the clinician serves as a resource teacher and assists the student with self-directed programming. In such cases, a standard school form is generally used. Clinicians interested in this type of programming should work with school administrators to refine or develop procedures consistent with school policy.

♦ STEPS IN NEGOTIATING A CONTRACT

Identifying Areas for Modification

The clinician and student together decide which of the areas relevant to voice need attention: respiration, phonation, resonance, interpersonal/psychological factors, lifestyle/high risk factors. Initially, the results of the diagnostic evaluation are presented in a factual manner by the clinician, who necessarily assumes the leadership role in interpreting assessment data. Since this is observable data and conclusions can be supported by evaluation results, targets usually emerge logically and with mutual acceptance by both parties.

Ordering Targets

Open discussion that results in reciprocal, rather than asymmetrical, input is critical at this stage of contract negotiation. The clinician, who will have professional insights drawn from experience and specialized training, may be predisposed to select a particular hierarchy of targets. However, the student's self-knowledge must be allowed equal weight in the negotiation process. The clinician can benefit from thoroughly exploring the student's perceptions and priorities, and in so doing, can encourage the student's participation in the therapy process.

It is imperative that a speech-language pathologist explain each of the targets and what is required in modifying each behavior. This should be done in a way that does not coerce a student to select a predetermined target. The speech-language pathologist should avoid using technical language that might confuse or intimidate a student and should avoid leading the student to "feed back" the clinician's own biases. Since the targets were mutually agreed on in the previous step of contract negotiation, a speech-language pathologist should be comfortable with allowing a student to sequence them.

Matching Targets and Approaches

Concurrent or Sequential

As the clinician and student observe the number and sequence of targets, patterns for attacking the modification process emerge. Some targets may form the basis for modification of future targets, whereas other targets may lend themselves to a concurrent approach. It is important to negotiate with the student how many targets will be undertaken at one time. Frequently, a student may be motivated to attack a large number of targets. However, if the student's semester schedule is heavy, as in seasonal sports participation, it may be judicious to contract the heavy commitment for the following semester and limit targets for the present semester. Frustration and failure may be inevitable for the student who is allowed to contract an unrealistic number of goals.

Acquisition of Facts and Information

At this stage of contract negotiations, the clinician presents a list of resources and techniques available for acquiring information and the student selects those that are most appealing (Table 4–1). For example, some students may prefer approaches that require little

TABLE 4-1.
Resources and Techniques for Acquiring Information

♦ readings	♦ library searches	♦ projects
♦ models (e.g., larynx)	♦ computers	♦ discussions
♦ observations	♦ group reports	♦ presentations
♦ tapes or films	♦ experiments	♦ field trips
♦ interviews	♦ lectures	

interpersonal communication (e.g., library searches, computer projects), whereas others may enjoy approaches that require more interaction (e.g., discussions, interviews, observations). Of course, interpersonal interaction will be a prime ingredient of later voice therapy stages, but at this stage, allowing a student to express preferences builds momentum by enhancing early learning.

Table 4-1 contains a list of resources and techniques could be used by a student as a preferential checklist. It may be necessary for the speech-language pathologist to describe the application of some of these resources so that a student can make informed choices.

Format for Implementation

The ASHA Task Force Report on Traditional Scheduling Procedures in Schools (Jones, Austin, MacLean, & Warkomski, 1973) acknowledged that special problems arise with scheduling at the secondary school level. It stated that students at the middle and high school levels usually have inflexible schedules. It recommended consideration of regularly scheduled speech-language classes as part of the academic curriculum.

Van Hattum (1969) stated that scheduling at the middle and high school levels is usually best accomplished on a two-visits-per-week basis. Battle and Van Hattum (1982) noted that problems with scheduling during the school day include students' unwillingness to miss classes. Frequently, the length of a voice therapy session does not coincide with the length of an academic class. Neidecker (1980) said, "High school students who may be able to assume more responsibility for themselves may need only one 1-hour-session per week" (p. 119). However, little research has been conducted concerning the effect of scheduling in the secondary schools.

The ASHA Task Force report (Jones et al., 1973) suggested that when there are severe scheduling conflicts, intensive services can be provided during the summer. Offering services in the late afternoons, evenings, or on Saturdays has also been suggested (O'Toole & Zaslow, 1969). For instance, some school corporations have included extended-hour services for secondary school students. Such programming may involve speech-language pathologists' work days being rearranged to include four 10-hour-days rather than five 8-hour-days. Speech-language pathologists may need to work with school administrators to develop flexible scheduling alternatives to traditional models.

Discussing available time and scheduling preferences with a student is usually valuable. For example, some students prefer intensive, short-term commitments. An all-day workshop, perhaps held on a Saturday or on an in-service day, combined with periodic follow-up, may be an appropriate format to adopt. Other adaptations include brown-bag lunch meetings once a week, evening tutorials, or after-school scheduling.

When therapy is conducted after school hours, the speech-language pathologist will need to negotiate the issue of "comp time" with school administrators. Of course, the speech-language patholo-gist working at the secondary school level should discuss the feasibil-ity of adopting alternative scheduling models with school adminis-trators before suggesting such variations to a student.

When voice therapy is conducted during the academic day, there are variations that can make the scheduling more meaningful for the adolescent. McKinley and Lord-Larson (1985) strongly advocated the use of course credit, because students invest at least as much time and energy in communication retraining as they do in other courses. A contract may provide useful documentation if a school system elects to offer an academic grade and course credit upon successful competi-tion of the contract. The voluntary nature of this system often seems to contribute to its success.

Another option for scheduling is to provide voice modification or professional voice training as an elective at the beginning of a school semester. Such a system involves considerable planning on the part of the speech-language pathologist. In-service training for school guidance counselors and advisors is particularly important, since they may be helpful in identifying students who might profit from a speech-language elective. This format is similar to a delivery of service model presented by Albritton (1984), who described the development of middle school language classes that were alternatives to the traditional "pull out of class" method of scheduling speech-language therapy.

It is especially important for a student to participate in setting up attendance criteria so that the expectations concerning attendance are explicitly stated and mutually agreed on. The contract might include a specific number of sessions or hours of programming. In such cases, absences would extend the duration of therapy so that the total number of sessions or hours would be completed. To avoid infrequent attendance, a percentage attendance criterion could be set in advance. Failure to achieve criterion (without adequate excuse) would result in termination or renegotiation of the contract.

Designing the implementation format involves a great deal of flexibility and creativity on the part of the student and speech-language pathologist. Areas that should be addressed include frequency and length of contacts with the speech-language pathologist, type of contact (e.g., individual therapy, group therapy, consultation/monitoring), course credit or noncredit, setting for therapy meetings, and attendance criteria.

Establishing Methods for Monitoring and Evaluating Progress

It is beneficial for students to realize the importance of monitoring vocal behaviors on a continuing basis and to understand milestones that indicate progress. The process of selecting evaluation procedures helps students gain a realistic perspective of what lies ahead. Discussions of these procedures also helps a clinician understand more about a student's personal style. However, a clinician should encourage students to try as many ways of monitoring and evaluating as possible. Some of the strategies that can provide feedback to students include tapes, videos, logs, diaries, checklists, graphs, percentages, reports from other sources, and oral self-reports. Although continual monitoring and evaluation are integral parts of the voice therapy process, scheduled documentation of progress can focus both the clinician and student on what has been accomplished and what tasks still lie ahead.

The reader is referred to Brodnitz's (1963) categories for determining the outcome of vocal rehabilitation, Boone's (1974) five dismissal criteria for voice patients, and Cooper's (1977) criteria for completing voice therapy. Cooper (1977) suggested using the laryngologist's report on visual impressions, the student and pathologist's evaluation of auditory characteristics, and the student's own sensory judgments. Depending on the lifestyle and aspirations of the individual, the standard for dismissal may not be complete rehabilitation. For instance, one student may be satisfied if most undesirable features (both attitudinal and behavioral) have been eliminated. Another student, who has a high investment in vocal performance (e.g. drama or choir), may strive for higher levels of proficiency.

A time limit for voice therapy can increase the efficient use of both the student and clinician's time and allay the fears of students who feel that enrollment in therapy is a "life sentence." Berryman

(1986) stated that voice therapy is typically of shorter duration than therapy for other speech-language problems. She noted that the time needed to change one vocal parameter is roughly equivalent to the time needed to change one speech sound. Voice therapy can proceed rapidly with a highly motivated adolescent, since much can be accomplished by the student independently. However, some students require a great deal of help with attitudinal and behavioral modification of vocal symptoms.

We have found that approximately 15 hours is a realistic amount of intervention time for an initial contract. This timeline prevents a student from thinking that change can occur without effort and allows sufficient time for in-depth programming. The contract can be renegotiated after 15 hours for complicated problems. In the case of less complicated vocal problems, dismissal prior to the contracted time results in positive attitudes toward the speech-language program.

The final phase of contract negotiation is determining the method for follow-up after direct intervention ceases. An advantage of discussing maintenance procedures is that a student gains a realistic understanding of the various stages of the rehabilitation process and an understanding that responsibilities continue, though in different form, after an acceptable level of proficiency has been reached. Techniques for follow-up and the dates and frequency of post-therapy checks should be addressed during this phase. Follow-up techniques include the clinician's evaluation of spontaneous speech (face-to-face, tape recordings, telephone calls), the student's self-evaluation, voice evaluation by peers and significant adults (casual or structured), and progress notes, letters, and checklists from the student and from teachers, parents, and peers. (Peers who have been part of the student's therapy group are especially good trained listeners.)

It should be remembered that behavioral changes of any kind are difficult to achieve. An individual's readiness to change is related to self-concept, to knowledge about what is involved, and to scheduling demands. Sometimes a clinician expects all students with voice problems to enroll in voice therapy and follow through until their problems are solved. However, a clinician must be flexible enough to alter expectations according to a student's input. Rather than being frustrated by a limitation imposed by the client, a clinician should be challenged to focus on achieveable goals. It is important to realize that the process of self-knowledge can continue even during times when there is no direct intervention. A short therapy segment may be a springboard for increased determination and commitment. Dismissal does not always have to be tied to total rehabilitation.

The therapeutic relationship may be marked by periods of intense interaction interspersed with periods during which a student deals with problems independently. This type of model can foster independence and self-growth and can enhance a student's motivation. It cannot be assumed that a student who "drops out" for a while is unmotivated. The priorities of a speech-language pathologist and an adolescent may not coincide in the short run, but may converge in the long run. The ability to adapt to changing needs and lifestyle demands can be demonstrated by a willingness to accept the student's right to self-determination.

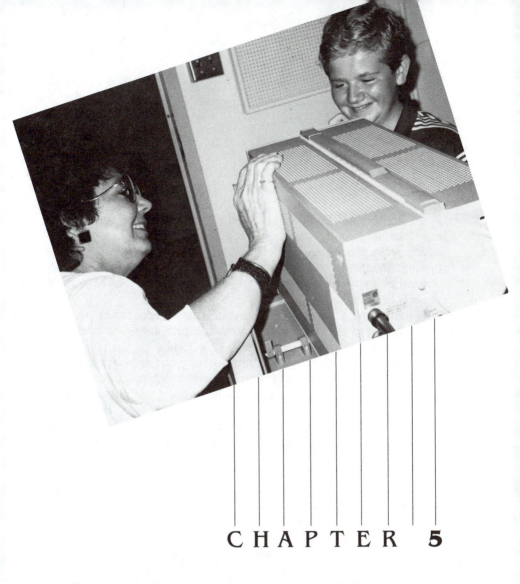

C H A P T E R **5**

The Therapeutic Process

In voice therapy, long-term goals (the expected outcome) and short-term goals (the prerequisite steps leading to the long-term goal) are usually written in behavioral terms. However, the establishment of a trusting therapeutic relationship is the foundation on which modification of vocal behavior is built, even though it cannot be defined precisely in behavioral terms.

Establishing a trusting relationship with an adolescent is sometimes a challenging task. Students are frequently uneasy with authority figures or adults they think may seek to change their behavior. Frequently, an adolescent may come to voice therapy with negative expectations or feelings that seem to put the speech-language pathologist at an immediate disadvantage. To dispel these preconceived mental sets, the speech-language pathologist must consider factors that contribute to the development of a warm, trusting relationship. Many of these factors are, of course, relevant to all relationships; others have particular significance to working with adolescents.

♦ PERSONAL ADJUSTMENTS BY THE CLINICIAN

The clinician working with adolescents must make conscious personal adjustments in attitudes (communicated both verbally and nonverbally), in the environment, and in the choice of materials. Attitudes toward the teenager can be conveyed through the use of posture, eye contact, intonation patterns, and vocabulary. Assuming a relaxed attitude that promotes a nonauthoritarian, friendly climate (such as placing both the clinician and student's chairs on the same side of a table) is usually helpful. Direct eye contact and a balance of clinician-student talking and listening times can promote an atmosphere of equality. It is sometimes difficult for a speech-language pathologist who has been working with young children to switch to more adult patterns. However, it is degrading for a young adult to hear exaggerated intonation patterns, such as are frequently used with young children. The use of plural pronouns, such as, "Now what did we do for homework this week?" and the excessive use of "should" statements ("You should do this or that") are also perceived negatively by older students. Because of their greater cognitive skills, adolescents can understand advanced terminology and explanations. Since the adolescent is sensitive to immature approaches, the speech-language pathologist should allow a student to take a leadership role (e.g., record keeping, note-taking) whenever possible.

The room in which voice therapy takes place should reflect the age and interests of the adolescent. If the room is used by a large number of students of different ages, it is important to have a corner that reflects more adult interests and is equipped with adult-sized furniture and decorations. Even the use of elementary school lined paper for note-taking should be avoided.

Clinicians often try to adapt materials used with elementary children for use with middle and high school students. However, experience sugggests this is usually obvious to the older student. Designing new materials specific to the adolescent population can avoid inadvertently insulting the teenager's emerging sense of maturity. The extra effort required is more than offset by the stimulation that results from working on a higher cognitive and experiential level. For example, the higher reading levels of adolescent students make it possible to utilize a wider range of reading materials. Adolescents also possess the skills necessary to share responsibility in identifying available resources and using audiovisual equipment.

Advances in technology have made many pieces of electronic equipment readily available and within the budgets of both students and school corporations. The speech-language pathologist should exploit this availability. For example, data collection can include use of Polaroid cameras and mini-tape recorders. Daily logs and record keeping are efficiently handled on computers. Graphics software is available to expedite the presentation of data, and students can use "Walkmans" to listen to voice therapy homework assignment tapes at their convenience. Adapting the classroom environment and materials to the adolescent can increase the student's motivation, the clinician's stimulation, and the sharing, creative atmosphere of the therapeutic interaction.

It might be helpful to remember some of the major differences between working with elementary-aged children and the adolescent population. Some of these differences are outlined in Table 5–1. Clinical experience suggests that the amount of voice therapy time devoted to behavior modification tasks is greater with younger children, whereas insight development requires a greater percentage of time with adolescents. Ideally, adolescent students assume greater responsibility for rehabilitation progress than younger children do. A therapy sequence designed for use with adolescents appears in Table 5-2.

TABLE 5-1.

How Voice Therapy with Adolescents Is Different from Voice Therapy with Younger Children

Children	Adolescents
Wants to please teacher.	Complicated, ambivalent feelings about authority figures.
Influenced by parental support of therapy program.	Wants independence from parents in therapy program.
Extrinsic reinforcement usually effective (stickers, tokens, praise, treats).	Intrinsic reinforcement usually effective, (individualized with reference to self-image, peer interactions, lifestyle activities).

Definition of goals:
  Major contributors: clinician, parents, teacher
  Minor contributor: student.
	Definition of goals:
	  Major contributors: student, clinician
	  Minor contributors: school personnel, parents.

Homework assignments structured (speech books), tangible (worksheets). Parents and teachers frequently involved.	Homework assignments relevant to a variety of situations, activities. Occasional involvement of school personnel, infrequent parental involvement.
Group therapy frequently provides competition, reinforcement, stimulated discussion. Clinician assumes major leadership role.	Individual therapy provides effective format for counseling, contracting. Group therapy provides important peer support. Clinician assumes indirect leadership role.
Referral to voice program: clinician parent, classroom teacher, physician.	Referral to voice program: counselors, advisors, nurse, physician, self-referrals.
Scheduling: students seen as frequently as possible in relatively short sessions.	Scheduling: students seen less frequently but for longer sessions. Intensive sessions and independent work supplementary.
Self-awareness and self-monitoring must be taught, reactions of others must be specifically defined.	Self-consciousness and awareness of peer group provide framework for discussion and analysis.
Concepts basic to voice program require significant therapy time.	Concepts basic to voice program require less time because of higher cognitive level.*
Materials generally concrete, action-oriented, visually appealing.	Complexity and scope of materials reflects social and cognitive development, age.
Balance between counseling and skill development: major amount of time spent practicing skills.	Balance between counseling and skill development: major amount of time spent in counseling or on insight producing tasks that are immediately applicable to situations, lifestyle.

*Applies to children without developmental disabilities.

TABLE 5-2.

A Sample Therapy Sequence for Adolescents

Developing the student's internal motivation

A. Elicit information about the student

B. Identify aspects of lifestyle where communication is important

C. Identify positive or satisfying aspects of current communication behavior

Defining the problem

A. Identify situations where vocal behavior has not met expectations

B. Review vocal behavior in terms of current needs and future goals

C. Review vocal behavior in terms of reactions of others (family, friends, teachers)

D. Target aspects of vocal behavior that student would/would not like to change

E. Interpret diagnostic results

F. Describe intervention options

Negotiating the contract (where applicable)

Analyzing the problem

A. Student acquires knowledge
   1. Scientific principles: normal vocal production, student's vocal production
   2. Interpersonal communication styles: general principles, analysis of others, self-analysis
   3. Lifestyle factors: general principles, self-analysis
B. Student demonstrates knowledge
   1. Describes vocal symptoms accurately
   2. Describes physiological factors affecting voice
   3. Describes psychosocial factors affecting voice

Defining characteristics of new and old behaviors

A. Explain when, how, and why inappropriate behaviors are used

B. Determine ways to avoid or change inappropriate behaviors

C. Determine alternative strategies to substitute for inappropriate behaviors

Producing short utterances with facilitating techniques

A. Produces target behavior in isolation
   1. Instruction, cues, model
   2. Instruction, cues
   3. Instruction
B. Prolongs/repeats target behavior
C. Stops/starts target behavior at will
D. Demonstrates both appropriate and inappropriate behaviors

(continued)

TABLE 5-2. *(continued)*

E. Produces target behavior, varying length of utterance
   1. Isolated sounds
   2. Syllables
   3. Words: lists, sentence completions, fill in the blanks, structured repertoire of responses, associations, responses to questions, word-generating activities
   4. Phrases: lists, salutations, expansion with adjectives/adverbs, rhymes, phrase completions, rewording (e.g., negatives, opposites)
F. Monitors and self-corrects each target level with accuracy
   1. Clinician identifies correct/incorrect production
   2. Clinician and student discuss characteristics of correct/incorrect production
   3. Student identifies specific techniques/cues that facilitate correct target production
   4. Student analyzes why and how these techniques/cues facilitate correct production
   5. Clinician and student devise data-keeping methods to determine accuracy

Producing Long Utterances of Increasing Complexity

A. Written text materials
   1. Sentences
   2. Paragraphs: limericks/jokes, verses/poetry, personally relevant materials, narrations/characterizations, dramatic readings
B. Visually-cued materials: sentences generated from pictures, sentence clusters generated from picture sequences
C. Verbally-cued materials: definitions, story completions, paraphrases/summaries, supporting evidence, refutations, role-playing
D. Self-generated materials: jokes, anecdotes, moral dilemmas, mini-debates, improvisations, extemporaneous speeches, recaps (sporting, social events), reviews/critiques (books, performances)
E. Monitors and self-corrects each target level (with standards)
   1. Clinician and student devise performance standards
   2. Clinician and student devise sampling techniques; percentage of session to analyze, tapes/videos/peers, interruption vs. post-hoc analysis, independent vs. joint analysis of responses
   3. Clinician and student analyze effect of length and context on performance
   4. Clinician and student devise preparatory sets and cues to facilitate correct production
   5. Clinician devises method for checking reliability of student's monitoring skills
   6. Clinician and student devise short-term and long-term record keeping systems

Habituation

A. Identify situations in student's everyday life that student would like to target (e.g., academic, social, recreational, family)

B. Design a sequence of rehearsal and practice activities analogous to those encountered in student's everyday life
C. Role-play simulated situations in voice therapy room
D. Analyze factors impeding appropriate vocal behavior: emotional/physical state, size/type of group, location, background noise, time of day
E. Role-play difficult situations with distractions present: visual, auditory, physical/motor, social/emotional
F. Student uses appropriate behaviors in selected situations for short durations (outside therapy)
G. Student records and analyzes performance: anecdotal records, checklists, logs, charts
H. Student uses appropriate behaviors in complex situations for extended periods of time
I. Evaluate student's general performance level
J. Compares student's behavioral and attitudinal progress in terms of established timelines for treatment
K. Confer with student on progress and revise, renegotiate, or project dismissal accordingly
L. Identify techniques for maintenance of correct behaviors: coping strategies, self-reinforcements, insights, acceptance of help from supportive others, recognition of secondary gains
M. Student uses appropriate behaviors in nontargeted situations
N. Student monitors and adjusts behavior without support from others.

♦ PERSONAL ADJUSTMENTS BY THE ADOLESCENT

Therapy with the adolescent requires a meshing of goals related to both skill acquisition and self-actualization. The process of self-actualization during adolescence includes goals such as:

♦ Accepting responsibility for changing vocal behavior
♦ Understanding self in relation to authority figures, family, peers, institutions, and social groups
♦ Understanding the effect of emotions on the reactions of self and others
♦ Improving decision-making skills by recognizing and evaluating options and resources and by projecting short- and long-term consequences of decisions
♦ Refining and enhancing self-esteem by developing confidence through responsible problem solving

When adolescents habituate vocal behaviors that are self-defeating and counterproductive, they need to understand not only the situations and events that trigger negative behaviors, but also their own cognitive coding. For example, Mary was so anxious in large group situations that she found it impossible to initiate conversations and spoke inaudibly when others approached her. She needed to understand her belief that others would not be interested in listening to her. Rather than telling herself that she had nothing to offer that was of interest to others, she had to learn to foster more positive internal statements concerning her own worth. Her sequence of insights proceeded in the following way:

1. Identify self-defeating behaviors and the situations in which they occur
2. Recognize erroneous assumptions and negative internal statements about self in high-risk situations
3. Understand how negative beliefs lead to self-defeating behaviors
4. Develop more positive assumptions
5. Practice (through trial, error, and analysis) new vocal behaviors consistent with positive assumptions concerning self
6. Practice conversational strategies for focusing attention on the interests and needs of others

Some students need guidance to understand that feelings may be suppressed and that even suppressed feelings can affect vocal behavior. They can then understand that awareness of feelings helps to gain control over them and that such control can enable a person to modify vocal behavior.

Self-examination (understanding of the student's attitudes towards, and reactions to significant others) and situational and contextual awareness (understanding surrounding circumstances and reinforcing events that support present behaviors) provide the tools to monitor behavior.

Sometimes insights emerge gradually and at other times they are discovered suddenly. Insights that are most relevant to vocal behavior are those related to how one views oneself, how one is viewed by others, feelings experienced on occasions when vocal anxieties are highest, and how interpersonal behavioral patterns conform to expectations of self and others.

◆ FACTORS RELATED TO SUCCESSFUL INTERVENTION

Neal's (1986) discussion of motivation and attendance underscores the clinical impression that these related factors seem to be of equal importance to the success of intervention with adolescents.

Boone (1977) noted the advantage of working with self-referred adolescents, and Neidecker (1980) reported that vocational choice may provide incentives to change communication patterns. Goda (1970) referred to the social needs and interests of adolescents and commented that they seemed more likely to be self-motivated than younger students. It may be that increased maturity provides the perceptual and cognitive skills to analyze cause and effect relationships appropriately. Greater involvement in dating and social activities may also lead the adolescent to conclude that changes in vocal behavior will have a positive effect on social relationships.

Neal (1976) and Bradford, Hosea, and Neal (1977) identified the factors most important for intervention success at the secondary level as being (1) consistent student attendance, (2) a student's motivation for self-improvement, and (3) a student's opinions of other people's attitudes toward the communication problem. Neal (1976) also discussed the decreasing role of parents and classroom teachers in therapy as a child grows older. He indicated, however, that their attitudes continue to influence the intervention process.

As children enter adolescence, the adult's perception of the student must change dramatically. This is fundamental both to the adult's understanding of the voice therapy program and to the roles the adult and student are assigned in the process. The speech-language pathologist's philosophy concerning intervention, the teacher's philosophy of education, and the parent's definition of the parent-child relationship must be markedly different with the teenage population than with younger children. The adolescent is in a stage of transition. The process of becoming an independent, responsible adult requires that the roles of authority figures be radically redefined. That is not to say that adult roles become less important, but that they are different.

According to Neal (1976), next to correction of a speech-language problem, the most frequently stated reason for dismissal from voice therapy is lack of motivation. Speech-language pathologists may wonder if poor motivation is sometimes the result of inappropriately designed therapy programs. The student's perception of the attitudes of others was ranked third in importance on Neal's (1976) survey and is highly relevant to both motivation and attendance. Fear or embarrassment at being singled out for help may trigger avoidance reactions, which include denial that a problem exists, rejection of the possibility that voice therapy could be helpful, and rebellion against suggestions that services be sought. School personnel and parents need to be aware of the way their actions and suggestions can communicate their attitudes toward a student and the use of resources. Well-meaning adults sometimes confront adolescents with statements such as, "I notice you've got something wrong with your voice. You should go see the speech-language pathologist to help you with your problem." This choice of language communicates negative feelings that will probably elicit embarrassment and defensiveness. It may be more advantageous to emphasize a student's own problem-solving abilities with statements such as, "What are your thoughts about taking advantage of some of the resources we have available here at school? For example, did you know we have a speech-language pathologist who knows a lot about voice? You might want to explore that opportunity."

♦ **CLINICIAN-STUDENT INTERACTION**

A clinician's attitude toward a student is revealed through body language, such as posture, gesture, and eye contact and through metalinguistic aspects, such as tone of voice, loudness level, and inflection. It may seem trite to say that if a clinician is relaxed, warm, and accepting, a student will be more at ease. However, the ways in which a clinician attends, listens, encourages, and focuses on information can be critical to the success of voice therapy.

Attending behaviors encourage a student to verbalize ideas and feelings. Active listening has a strong reinforcing effect. It is often helpful if a clinician refrains from adding to the student's meaning. Confirming comments, such as "I can understand what you went through" or "That seems a helpful insight" may allow the student to explore further and to feel a sense of increased responsibility.

If, however, a student rambles or digresses, selective inattention may be a useful technique to return the student to a more productive track. Selective inattention strategies are usually nonverbal signs. For example, a student who is telling stories when the clinician feels it may be more productive to discuss how the student feels now, may observe that the clinician seems attentive when the discussion is about feelings and seems inattentive when the discussion is about past events. Inattentive behaviors may include looking at the clock or looking out the window.

Verbal strategies that help a clinician guide productive verbalization include paraphrasing, clarifying, and perception-checking. Paraphrasing is used to test the clinician's perception of what has been said. Generally, the clinician rephrases and summarizes the student's message when there is a natural break in the conversation. When paraphrasing is used successfully, the student usually provides a confirming response or other cue indicating that the clinician's understanding is accurate.

If a message has been confusing, the speech-language pathologist may seek clarification by probing (e.g., "I'm not sure I understand. Can you tell me more?"). These remarks should be phrased to elicit clearer statements from a student without implying that the student is confused. It is important that the speech-language pathologist refrain from interpreting or explaining. Requests for illustrations or repetition are the best ways of clarifying the student's ideas and feelings.

Similarly, asking for feedback from a student is a technique used to check the accuracy of the clinician's listening skills. The technique of "perception-checking" involves both the giving and receiving of information concerning the accuracy of a perception. For example, statements such as "I want you to tell me if I'm understanding exactly what you mean" can lead into a paraphrase of what the clinician thinks the student has said. This allows the student to correct the clinician and suggests confidence in the student's abilities.

A clinician should be sensitive to a student's readiness to accept feedback, because frequent unsolicited opinions may cause resistance, resentment, or denial. Feedback should not consist of personal judgments and should focus on behavior and issues an adolescent is capable of changing. Feedback should be a prompt response to specific behavior, and should be given in small amounts so that attention can be fully focused on manageable items.

Developing skills to encourage a student to respond openly is important for clinicians working with adolescents. These skills are frequently referred to as "leading" and require anticipating the direction of a student's thoughts and responding with encouraging statements. The goals of leading are to help a student explore and elaborate on statements, to explore a variety of options and freely discuss alternatives, and to encourage a student to be involved in and maintain responsibility for decisions.

Indirect comments such as "Tell me why you are here" or "What do you think this means?" encourage a student to elaborate. Pauses or "expectant looks" can also serve as indirect leads. A speech-language pathologist should always have a clear purpose for a lead, make the lead general, and pause long enough for a student to respond.

A clinician tries to focus a discussion with direct leads. Statements such as "Can you give me an example of what happens to cause you to feel that way?" or "Tell me some more about how your friend reacted to your new voice" generally help a student to elaborate. A clinician can also help focus a discussion with leads such as "What word or words can best describe what you've been telling me?" and "What were your feelings as we talked?" It is important that a clinician clearly verbalize a lead.

Most leads are in question form, and it is important that they be open-ended so that they cannot be answered merely with "yes" or "no" responses. Generally, questions beginning with "how," "what," or "why" will result in more elaborated responses.

"Reflecting" lets a student know that the clinician is perceiving an issue from the student's viewpoint. Successful reflecting requires identifying a student's feelings, reading nonverbal body language for implied feelings, and paraphrasing a student's message. The clinician should use language appropriate to the student's intellectual level and cultural experiences. Guard against using the same opening leads, and include nonverbal responses, such as head-nodding, that can prevent segmenting a discussion with too many verbal responses.

When summarizing an interview, a clinician should leave the student with the feeling that progress has been made. The clinician may decide to state the summary or may ask the student to provide a summary. It is important that no new ideas or information be introduced during a summary so that an interview does not end with unexplored topics. Summarizing can also be used at the beginning of a therapy session, when a summary of the previous session can provide continuity for the new session.

Clinicians must understand their own emotional reactions during therapy sessions. They must decide if their responses are related to their own personal experiences or to what a student is saying. They must then decide if sharing their feelings with the student would be productive to the goals of the session.

Speech-language pathologists should be aware that they will not be capable of working with all of the issues or feelings that can surface during voice therapy sessions. Students may need to be referred to other specialists. Caution should be used in exploring the feelings of students who have personality problems, who are under pressure, or who have difficulty dealing with emotions. Speech-language pathologists may want to avoid emotional issues if they doubt their abilities to deal with such issues, if support services are inadequate or time is limited, or if the school or a student's parents discourage the exploration of feelings.

◆ *RECOGNITION OF STUDENTS' LEARNING STYLES*

An analysis of learning styles serves as a reminder that people think and learn in different ways. Content will make more sense to a student if it is presented in a manner consistent with the student's preferred style of learning. Speech-language pathologists who have thought about their own preferred learning styles are less likely to impose those styles on adolescents.

Bramson and Bramson (1985) proposed five categories of learning styles: synthetic, idealistic, pragmatic, analytic, and realistic. Their research showed that only about 15 percent of people use the five styles equally, 50 percent have a single preferred style, and the remaining 35 percent use a combination of styles.

Some students need to think and talk a great deal about different ways of solving problems. Bramson and Bramsom (1985) would describe such individuals as "synthesist thinkers." It's ideas that make a difference to these students, not facts. In working with the synthesist, the speech-language pathologist should assume the role of the practical person without detracting from the student's enthusiasm and should remember that the synthesist sees arguments as fun, not as confrontations. The synthesist will probably enjoy the process of contrasting different treatment ideas. Although the speech-language pathologist may feel a need to encourage the synthesist to target concrete solutions, allowing the student time to develop insights may result in a greater commitment to the treatment program.

Idealists, on the other hand, are usually concerned with goals, ethics, and mutually agreed-on views. They enjoy focusing on similarities, pursuing agreement, and identifying with explanations involving what is good for them and others. These students would probably enjoy reading about links between nutrition and physical well-being, the effects of drugs on the mind and body, and the physiology of a well-functioning system. They may be ideal candidates for clear-cut definitions of behavioral objectives linked to their overall vocational and educational goals. Since idealists often feel guilty about their imperfections, the speech-language pathologist should ensure that short-term rewards for gains are present as well as long-term rewards. Sufficient praise and careful documentation of progress can offset discouragement when larger goals are not met rapidly. An idealist can become so committed to the goals of good vocal hygiene that this commitment can be used as a positive force in peer support situations.

Pragmatists are concerned with getting things started immediately and not worrying too much about long-term planning. They are resourceful, innovative, and adaptable. However, enthusiasm sometimes lags if a project takes very long. Pragmatists can easily understand that their voices can be changed and will be eager to get started, but they may not want to waste time discussing a detailed treatment approach. The speech-language pathologist should capitalize on the pragmatist's enthusiasm for moving ahead by providing action-oriented assignments immediately, demonstrating flexibility, and reinforcing the student's action, energy, and commitment. Growth may occur best in an experience-based format rather than one focusing on theoretical insight. The speech-language pathologist should maintain a clear focus on a single goal so that a student does not undertake more than can be accomplished successfully. Demonstrations of success, summaries of progress, and the relevance of present tasks to the next step in the sequence will help maintain the student's momentum. Role-playing is an excellent strategy for this type of student, and motivation is highly correlated to the immediate demands of the student's lifestyle.

Analysts are concrete thinkers who give little weight to feelings. They believe in solving problems by patiently gathering data and carefully searching for the right solutions. They are concerned with thoroughness and accuracy, and may seem obsessive about small details. A speech-language pathologist should be prepared to commit a significant amount of time to analyzing such a student's voice, discussing various remediation theories, providing additional readings, and developing a hierarchical sequence of goals. Praise from the speech-language pathologist may seem irrelevant to these students since reinforcement comes from grappling with issues. The speech-language pathologist should provide the analyst with information, careful referencing, and a variety of theoretical perspectives and should allow the student to assume a major role in organizing materials, summarizing information, and structuring the hierarchy of therapy goals. The evolution of a carefully orchestrated therapy program is rewarding in itself for the analyst. An analytic student may seem threatening to an inexperienced clinician, but exploiting the analyst's need for systemization can help the clinician work with these students.

Realists are most concerned about whether or not recommendations can be accomplished. They want to know, for example, how the voice can be changed and what recommendations can be implemented. They do not relate to fanciful or theoretical explanations or to too much detail, preferring facts, concrete examples of specific situations, and straightforward summaries. Such students distrust compromise, like to see their objectives clearly, and become impatient with soul-searching and analysis. The speech-language pathologist will need to be assertive, since realists have little respect for those they consider "soft," idealistic, or lacking in follow through. Realists are goal-oriented, so expected results should be spelled out concisely and unequivocally. The realist is an excellent observer, and therapy activities should draw on those observational skills and on the realists' desire for factual evidence of progress. For example, imitation of a variety of vocal behaviors and facilitating techniques and data keeping activities (charts, graphs, logs, workbooks, worksheets) would probably appeal to the realist. Realists are sensitive to inconsistency, appreciate a practical, no-nonsense approach to intervention, and value consistency and directness.

The categories used in the previous discussions are those of Bramson and Bramson (1985). It is not suggested that this categorization system is anything other than a convenient method of highlighting the fact that diversity exists in the way people think and learn. Other writers have suggested equally useful designations for thinking and learning styles. It is important to remember that no one individual fits neatly into a single category. However, clinicians should also remember that most students will have preferred learning styles and should be aware of how their own learning styles affect their expectations of student performance.

Students who feel they have some control over how and what they are learning develop an inner sense of satisfaction and mastery. They have the sense of pleasure that results from learning in a way that they help to determine rather than in a way that is forced on them. Choice, however, should not be equated with permissiveness. Permissiveness is allowing students to do whatever they want. Choice means combining structure and autonomy so that goals are clear, but the method for achieving the goals is flexible.

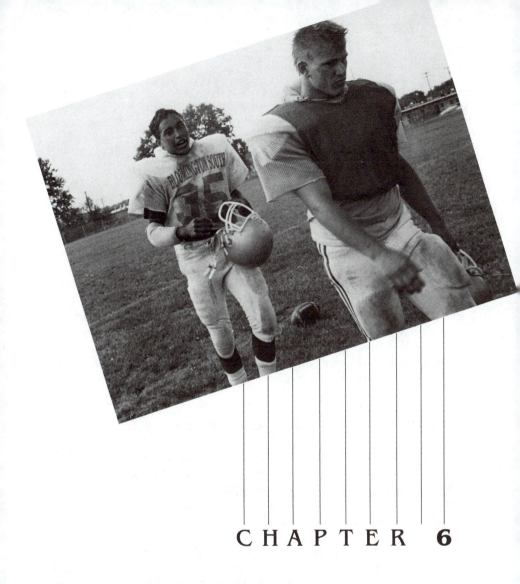

CHAPTER 6

Case Histories, Contracts, and Sample Program Plans

I n a holistic approach to programming, the student's vocal symptoms are considered and dealt with in the context of the individual's own perspective and lifestyle. To illustrate ways in which holistic voice programs are designed and implemented, some examples of case histories, contracts and program plans are presented. The adolescents selected for inclusion in this chapter are typical of students seen in the public school setting. The programs, however, are not intended to be viewed as model programs that can be transferred and applied to other individuals. Rather, they are examples of how diagnostic information was translated into programs that were effective for the specific needs of these particular students.

♦ TAMMY: AN EXAMPLE OF VOCAL ABUSE

Tammy, age 15, had been a member of the pompom squad for 2 years before earning a place on the varsity cheerleading squad of her high school. She was referred to the speech-language pathologist by the public speaking teacher because of frequent periods of hoarseness and occasional aphonia that made it difficult for her to participate in classroom speaking projects.

The teacher reported that Tammy seemed to find it difficult to control her urge to talk even when her voice was in "bad shape," and described her as an excitable, vivacious person. He observed that Tammy was constantly regaling her friends with stories and anecdotes, and noted that she could always be heard above the others in a group. Tammy had responded to his suggestions that she rest her voice more by saying that she didn't want to be seen as a "boring, mousy person."

Initially, Tammy reacted negatively to being referred to the speech-language pathologist, saying that "was just the way she was," that she knew many cheerleaders who sounded hoarse, and that many people found her raspy voice attractive. However, because the otolaryngology report showed the presence of bilateral vocal nodules, and because of her parent's concern, Tammy agreed to a trial period of voice therapy.

100

During subsequent discussions, it emerged that a significant part of Tammy's self-concept was tied to being "center stage." She viewed herself as being energetic, lively, and one who could lead and entertain. Since her grades were average, her recognition and status in school came not from academic achievement but from membership in groups that she perceived as having high social status.

Tammy engaged in a very demanding set of physical and vocal behaviors. Her schedule included enthusiastic participation in many physically exhausting activities, accompanied by loud talking, shrieking, and laughing. In the evenings, she spent hours on the telephone or invited friends to her home to work on homework assignments. Her record player was in constant use and she strained to talk over the background noise. She was frequently physically and emotionally "hyped-up" and rarely went to sleep before midnight. Late-night studying contributed to arguments with her parents that frequently ended in crying jags.

An outline and discussion of Tammy's voice therapy sequence follows.

Evaluation

I. Factors Precipitating Negative Behaviors
   A. Lifestyle
      1. Cheerleading and gymnastics practice after school
      2. Cheering at athletic events
      3. Loud singing and talking at social events
      4. Long telephone conversations with friends
      5. Late nights (fatigue)
II. Negative Behaviors Observed
   A. Chronic hoarseness and periodic aphonia
   B. Excessive amounts of vocalization
   C. Vocal impersonations
   D. Loud vocal level
   E. Hard glottal attacks
   F. Neck and facial tension
   G. Limited listening skills
   H. Denial of vocal problem
III. Sample Target Behaviors for Therapy
   A. Voice conservation techniques
   B. Modification of lifestyle and self-image
   C. Analysis of interpersonal skills, need satisfaction, and physical-emotional resources

Contract Negotiation

In negotiating a contract, the speech-language pathologist discussed with Tammy how her voice affects the successful achievement of her present and future goals. Tammy's only real concern was periodic aphonia. Therefore, voice conservation was of top priority. She agreed to analyze her interpersonal skills primarily, it seemed, because she wished to convince the speech-language pathologist that her personality and enthusiasm necessitated using her voice as she did. She vehemently refused to discuss significantly modifying her lifestyle because it "suited her just fine." Tammy's gregarious nature is reflected in her choice and ordering of the therapeutic goals.

I. Areas for Modification
   A. Phonation
   B. Interpersonal and psychological factors
   C. Lifestyle
II. Ordering Targets
   A. Conserve voice
   B. Analyze interpersonal skills
III. Matching Targets and Approaches
   A. Concurrent approach
   B. Acquisition of facts and information
      1. Discussions
      2. Projects
      3. Observations
      4. Group reports
      5. Interviews
      6. Lectures
      7. Experiments
      8. Field trips
      9. Models
IV. Format for Implementation
   A. Frequency and length of contact with speech-language pathologist: once per week for 45 minutes
   B. Type of contact: group
   C. Twenty percent course credit in lieu of one public speaking class per week based on her performance in group therapy
   D. Speech-language pathologist's office
   E. Ninety percent attendance (not more than two absences)

Therapy Plan

Since Tammy was reluctant to attend voice therapy, the speech-language pathologist decided to create an informal, more social atmosphere by having soft drinks available during the first session and arranging the chairs around a circular table. Two other students who also exhibited vocally abusive practices were attending weekly therapy with Tammy. During the next three therapy sessions, one student attended a private discussion with the speech-language pathologist while the other two students were assigned films or readings on vocal fold physiology in the library.

I. Developing the Student's Internal Motivation
   A. Share biographical, academic, extracurricular, social, and recreational information
   B. Students interview each other and develop lists of areas in their lives in which communication is important to them

II. Defining the Problem
   A. Attend an individual session of 15 minutes with the speech-language pathologist to review diagnostic results and discuss the goals and options for intervention
      1. Prepare a randomly-ordered list of positive and negative voice-use situations.
      2. Compare perceptions of self and others on ranking task and discuss possible targets for change.

III. Analyzing the Problem
   A. Share knowledge gained from library readings of normal vocal fold physiology by demonstrating with a model of the larynx.
   B. Speech-language pathologist explains and demonstrates effect of vocal abuse on larynx
   C. Videotape and replay group discussions of homework assignments to aid discussion and analysis of communication skills.
   D. Speech-language pathologist discusses lifestyle factors and how they affect voice production
      1. "Brain storming" session
      2. List lifestyle factors affecting members' own vocal behaviors
   E. Students present oral reports (midterm evaluation for progress report)
      1. Speech-language pathologist grades reports for accuracy and scope
      2. Group members provide feedback on oral presentaton style

IV. Defining Characteristics of New vs. Old Behaviors
   A. Summarize findings of audiotapes and logs from homework assignment (See IV-C-6)
   B. Discuss environmental controls and alternative voice strategies
      1. Reset volume control on stereo from 6 to 3
      2. Place timer near telephone and limit calls to 10 or 15 minutes
      3. Determine time in evening after which phone calls will not be accepted or made
      4. Allot quiet reading time before sleep

     5. Reduce length of homework sessions with friends

     6. Improve talking/listening ratio

     7. Reduce vocal impersonation

     8. Increase number of questions asked in social interactions

     9. Improve breath support for projected speech (e.g., cheerleading)

   10. Decrease tension in face and neck muscles

   11. Match loudness level to situational demands (increase soft talking)

   12. Identify times when it is pleasant to be alone (provide time for vocal rest)

  C. Outside assignments

     1. Identify four situations in which voice use is good

     2. Identify at least three situations in which voice use is poor

     3. Present a list of positive and negative voice use situations to one peer and one adult and ask each to rank-order the list according to their perceptions

     4. Read assigned information about interpersonal communication styles

     5. Observe communication styles and skills of television actors and admired adult friends

     6. Audiotape cheerleading practice session, telephone conversation, and homework session with friend

     7. Prepare daily log (including hours of sleep, bedtime, daily volume setting of record player, number of telephone calls per day, number and length of friends' visits

V. Methods for Monitoring and Evaluating Progress

  A. Tapes

  B. Videos

  C. Diaries

  D. Checklists

  E. Reports from other sources

  F. Self-reports (oral)

VI. Timelines for Treatment Schedule and Dismissal Criteria

  A. Level of proficiency to be achieved in each target area

     1. Voice conservation techniques

       a. Eliminate neck and facial tension (100 percent)

       b. Eliminate hard glottal attacks (85 percent)

       c. Eliminate vocal impersonations (100 percent)

       d. Decrease amount of vocalization (20 percent)

       e. Understand principles of vocal hygiene (95 percent)

     2. Analysis of interpersonal skills

       a. Data keeping on listening skills (100 percent accuracy)

     3. Favorable report from physician

B. Maximum duration of therapy; two semesters
C. Progress review
   1. Dates for progress report: midsemester and end of semester
   2. Persons to receive progress reports: parents, public speaking teacher, physician
   3. Date for termination, extension, or revision of treatment plan: end of each semester
D. Frequency and type of follow-up after cessation of therapy sessions
   1. Frequency: once a month for three months
   2. Techniques: evaluation of spontaneous speech in face-to-face or telephone interview
      a. Self-evaluation
      b. Public speaking teacher's evaluation of voice
      c. Physician's evaluation of status of vocal folds

◆ LAMONT: AN EXAMPLE OF ALLERGIC REACTIONS

Lamont, age 16, was referred to the speech-language pathologist by the school nurse who, while treating him for abrasions sustained during football practice, noticed that he exhibited audible wheezing and an extremely hoarse voice.

During questioning, Lamont stated that he was taking medication for hay fever. The case history revealed that Lamont had broken his nose as a child. Since then, he'd had difficulty breathing, especially during spring and fall, the hay fever seasons. His family reported that he breathed noisily during sleep. Lamont said he had used various over-the-counter preparations to try to "clear his head." He reported that his mouth was frequently dry and his throat hurt during football practices. He also reported that he frequently lost his voice during football calisthenics. Since Lamont reported that he had not been seen by a physician for this problem, the speech-language pathologist requested a medical evaluation.

The evaluation by the speech-language pathologist revealed that Lamont's respiration for speech was characterized by adequate depth of inspiration, but limited expiratory control. It was observed that Lamont habitually breathed through his mouth and assumed an open-mouth position at rest. Observation of the orofacial structures revealed a deviated nasal septum and puffiness and redness of the eyes. Redness of the faucial pillars was also observed. Lamont's voice was characterized by a raspy, hoarse quality with periodic aphonia on unstressed syllables. He said that his voice was "okay for an athlete" and it didn't bother him at all, he just wished he could breathe better.

His vocalization pattern was characterized by short, tense phrases interrupted by labored inhalations, so that the continuity and flow of speech was disturbed. He used a low pitch level, infrequent use of inflections, and frequent throat clearing. Lamont's tonal focus appeared to be toward the back of the throat with minimal articulatory movement visible. The resonance pattern was predominately hyponasal and the oral consonants /b,d,g/ were substituted for the nasal consonants /m,n,ŋ/.

Results of the medical examination showed edema and redness of the vocal folds and entire vocal tract. The otolaryngologist made a subsequent referral to an allergist who ascertained that Lamont was highly allergic to dust, mold, and pollen. Desensitization therapy was instituted by the allergist and Lamont was advised to refrain from using nonprescription medication. The allergist explained that some of the preparations that Lamont had used had caused swelling of the nasal mucosa that had exacerbated, rather than helped, the narrowing of the airway caused by the deviated septum. Additionally, these preparations had contributed to dryness of the vocal tract. This dryness and irritation, as well as the vocal attempts Lamont had adopted to compensate for his swollen vocal mechanism, had compounded the original problem.

An outline and discussion of Lamont's voice therapy sequence follows.

Evaluation

I. Factors Precipitating Negative Behaviors
  A. Medical
    1. Deviated nasal septum
    2. Alterations in respiratory tract due to allegic reactions
    3. Alterations in respiratory tract due to self-medication
    4. Limited fluid intake
  B. Vocal Compensations and Habits
    1. Throat clearing
    2. Strained vocalization
    3. Short phrasing of utterances
    4. Substitution of oral consonants for nasal consonants
  C. Lifestyle
    1. Frequent exposure to airborn allergies during outdoor football practice
    2. Frequent, prolonged vocal demands accompanying physical exertion (calisthenic chants)
    3. Self-concept highly related to perception of the "macho athlete"
II. Negative Behaviors Observed
  A. Limited expiratory control

B. Mouth-breathing
C. Raspy, hoarse voice quality
D. Discontinuity of rate and phrasing
E. Limited inflections
F. Minimal articulatory movements
G. Back tone focus
H. Hyponasal resonance

III. Sample Target Behaviors for Therapy
  A. Analysis of medical factors and vocal compensations
  B. Modification of abusive behaviors:
    1. Strain during calisthenics
    2. Throat clearing
    3. Allergy management
  C. Improvement of respiratory patterns
  D. Improvement of balance of oral/nasal resonance
    1. Forward tone focus
    2. Increased mouth opening
    3. Articulatory precision

Contract Negotiation

  I. Areas for Modification
  A. Respiration
  B. Resonance
  C. Lifestyle and high-risk factors
 II. Ordering Targets
  A. Analyze medical factors and vocal compensations
  B. Improve respiratory patterns
  C. Eliminate abusive behaviors
  D. Improve balance of oral/nasal resonance
III. Matching Targets and Approaches
  A. Sequential approach
  B. Acquisition of facts and information
    1. Medical illustrations and models
    2. Readings and medical references
    3. Explanations by speech-language pathologist
 IV. Format for Implementation
  A. Frequency and length of contact with speech-language pathologist
    1. Consultation and monitoring during football season (two 30-minute consultations followed by one 15-minute monitoring session per month)
    2. Two 20-minute sessions per week during spring semester
  B. Type of contact: individual

C. No credit for therapy

D. Therapy in speech-language pathologist's office

E. Two mandatory initial consultations, 90 percent attendance during spring semester

Therapy Plan and Implementation

Since Lamont's schedule and priorities were heavily influenced by his participation in the football program, he supported the speech-language pathologist's suggestion that the major therapy commitment take place during the spring semester. However, by scheduling two consultations during the fall, the speech-language pathologist was able to provide Lamont with some basic information and to monitor the effects of the new medications throughout the first semester.

I. Developing the Student's Internal Motivation

   A. Discuss effects of new medication on respiration and energy level, especially during participation in football and related activities.

   B. Describe breathing and vocal behaviors in terms of what is appropriate for an athlete (spring).

   C. Present and discuss results of homework assignment (fall and spring).

II. Defining the Problem

   A. Discuss situations where breathing and vocal behavior have not met expectations (fall).

   B. Project plans for what Lamont would like to be doing in 10 years and how breathing and current vocal behaviors may influence achievement of those goals (spring).

   C. Analyze tapes made in homework assignment (fall). (See IV-C-3)

   D. Review diagnostic results and student's perceptions of the problem (fall).

III. Analyzing the Problem

   A. Review upper respiratory tract structure and function:

      1. Types of obstruction

      2. Compensatons or adaptations

      3. Effective medication

      4. Mouth vs. nose breathing (advantages and disadvantages)

      5. Fluid intake and lubrication of the vocal tract

      6. The influence of nasal obstruction on articulation, resonance, and respiration

      7. Abusive practices and their effects

      8. Environmental irritants

   B. Present oral report on specific medical, chemical, environmental, and abusive factors influencing the consistency of

breathing and vocal symptoms.
IV. Defining Characteristics of New vs. Old Behaviors
  A. Develop format for charting frequency and severity of inappropriate behaviors and precipitating factors
  B. Review patterns precipitating inappropriate behaviors and devise alternative strategies
  C. Outside assignments
    1. Make list of sportcasters on TV and research to find out those who have been successful athletes (spring)
    2. Log times during football season and nonfootball season when respiration and voice do not interfere with performance (fall and spring)
    3. Record reading passage
      a. After football practice
      b. Immediately after awakening
      c. At a time when voice is "at its best" (fall)
  V. Methods for Monitoring and Evaluating Progress
  A. Logs
  B. Checklists
  C. Graphs
  D. Self-reports (oral)
  E. Quizzes
VI. Timelines for Treatment Schedules and Dismissal Criteria
  A. Level of proficiency to be achieved in each target area
    1. Analyze medical factors and vocal compensations (90 percent on quiz)
    2. Improve respiratory patterns (85 percent)
    3. Eliminate abusive behaviors (85 percent)
    4. Improve balance of oral/nasal resonance (75 percent)
  B. Maximum duration of therapy: two semesters
  C. Progress review
    1. Dates for progress report: first and last sessions of the spring semester.
    2. Persons to receive progress report: physician, school nurse, parents
    3. Date for termination, extension, or revision of treatment plan: end of the spring semester
  D. Frequency and type of follow-up after cessation of therapy sessions
    1. Frequency: once per month during the football season
    2. Techniques
      a. clinician's evaluation of spontaneous speech in face-to-face interview
      b. student's self-evaluation of breathing patterns

Discussion

Prolongation of /n, m, ŋ/ were practiced and timed to improve nasal resonance, forward tone focus, and the length and control of expiration. Cues included use of the See-Scape, feeling vibrations on the bones of the face, and the nasal emission of air. Lamont charted the number of repetitions on /n, m, ŋ/ on one exhalation (goal = 30). A variation of this activity was to hum pitch patterns of football chants, cadences, or tunes using /m/. Oral/nasal word pairs (See Appendix A) were used to practice and contrast kinesthetic and auditory cues. (For example, Lamont described that the words *be/me* were identical in all aspects except for the direct nasal resonance and nasal emission of air felt on /m/). Chanting words, phrases, and sentences containing nasal consonants provided the opportunity to emphasize and prolong nasal reverberations. Initially, it was easier for Lamont to maintain continuity of voicing throughout an entire word when the words did not contain plosives, stops, and unvoiced continuants. As he progressed, more phonetic complexity was introduced. (See Appendix A.)

A sporting theme was used when Lamont practiced word lists and phrases to capitalize on his interest in football. Lamont generated word lists based on topics such as states and cities (with nasal consonants) that had good football teams, and sports and sports-related terms ending in "ing." Practice materials at the "phrase" level included scores with numbers containing nasals, phrases heard at sporting events, and names of players and coaches containing nasal consonants. The sports theme was continued throughout the treatment plan. It had the advantage of encouraging some immediate carryover, since many of the phrases and sentences practiced were used in Lamont's daily conversations and activities. Lamont reported that when he was watching TV, he often got good ideas for words and phrases to use in his voice therapy program.

The sports theme also provided for integration of respiratory and resonance goals. For example, during the production of long, complex utterances involving descriptions of football plays, Lamont monitored not only the resonance characteristics, but also the appropriateness of respiratory patterns. Elimination of abusive behaviors and correct respiratory support for projected speech were also rehearsed in chants and cadences used during football practice and game situations. Reading materials were drawn primarily from sports magazines, school newspapers, and the sporting sections of city newspapers. Lamont frequently brought articles to voice therapy that he wanted to share with the speech-language pathologist. Lamont then used these articles to structure interviews to practice spontaneous speech.

♦ ESTHER: AN EXAMPLE OF PMS

Esther, age 16, requested an appointment with the speech-language pathologist. She was the captain of her high school debate team and described a problem with her voice that occasionally interfered with her performance in debate tournaments. She stated that her voice was usually clear and strong, but her voice had "really let her down" during some tournaments. Since she was very concerned about her record as a debater, she felt she could not afford being penalized by these voice fluctuations.

The speech-language pathologist could detect no problems in Esther's voice and suggested that Esther "drop in" to the office sometime when she perceived her voice as unacceptable.

When Esther returned two weeks later, the speech-language pathologist was startled by the extreme change in her voice quality. She exhibited severe hoarseness and hyponasality. The speech-language pathologist questioned Esther extensively concerning the possibility of the symptoms being related to a cold or allergic reaction. Esther's responses were intense. She said she definitely did not have a cold and that she had never had allergies in her life. When the speech-language pathologist gently indicated that it is sometimes difficult to identify the "trigger mechanisms" for allergic reactions, Esther became agitated and stated that her "chances of winning the upcoming debate were practically zero." Esther seemed so agitated and upset during the discussion, that the speech-language pathologist wondered if the problem was the result of emotional tension. However, the speech-language pathologist remembered that she had been impressed by Esther's calm and rational manner during their initial interview.

The speech-language pathologist hypothesized that Esther's intermittent symptoms might be related to reactions to allergens or reactions to stress (i.e., pressures surrounding debate tournaments) and asked Esther to keep a log of her activities. She was to note details concerning her daily routine, diet, moods, and voice symptoms. She was to return in two months for another conference with the speech-language pathologist. Esther was counseled in the interim concerning general principles of vocal hygiene and cautioned to avoid vocally abusive behaviors when symptoms were present.

When Esther's log was examined at the end of 8 weeks, the speech-language pathologist was surprised by the cyclical pattern of symptoms. For three days following the conference, Esther's log showed the presence of the following conditions: hoarseness, nasal stuffiness and congestion, sneezing, coughing, irritability, increased food consumption, fatigue, and eye irritations (unable to wear contact lenses to read debate notes). For the next three weeks, none of these symptoms were recorded. However, symptoms recorded during the fourth week were very similar to those noted above. The second month of the log reflected a pattern similar to that of the first month: three symptom-free weeks followed by a recurrence of symptoms.

The speech-language pathologist suspected a correlation between the vocal symptoms and Esther's menstrual cycle. She thought that Esther might be affected by premenstrual syndrome (PMS). To verify her impressions, the speech-language pathologist suggested that Esther consult a local medical authority with special interest in PMS. The speech-language pathologist told Esther to be sure to take her log and her calendar to show to the physician.

Results of the physician's report indicated that Esther's pattern of vocal symptoms was compatible with patterns associated with PMS. He explained that changes in the laryngeal and nasal mucosa are sometimes related to hormonal fluctuations. Therefore, the hoarse voice quality that occurred the week before the onset of menstruation was due to edema of the vocal folds. The hyponasality, occurring concurrently, was the result of obstruction of the nasal passages by similarly swollen tissue. The physician outlined several possible treatment strategies including changes in diet and medication. He also advocated continued consultation with the speech-language pathologist to ensure appropriate vocal hygiene during times when Esther's speech mechansim was vulnerable to vocal abuse.

An outline and discussion of Esther's voice therapy sequence follows.

Evaluation

I. Factors Precipitating Negative Behaviors
    A. Medical
        1. Cyclical swelling of nasal and laryngeal mucosa
    B. Lifestyle
        1. High expectations for personal performance
        2. Exacerbated anxiety and emotional lability during week preceding menstruation
        3. Prolonged, sustained speaking situations (debate tournaments and practice sessions)
    C. Interpersonal
        1. Premenstrual fatigue, irritability, and tension reduced effectiveness in interactions with debate team members
II. Negative Behaviors Observed
    A. Hyponasal resonance
    B. Hoarse laryngeal quality

    C. Effortful speaking style

    D. Vocal variety limited to loudness and pitch increase

    E. Lack of awareness of principles of vocal hygiene

    F. Vocally abusive behaviors (crying jags, loud emotional outbursts)

III. Sample Target Behaviors for Therapy

    A. Awareness of premenstrual changes and effects on voice

    B. Identification of physical symptoms associated with PMS

    C. Adaptation of lifestyle, where possible, to correlate with cyclical physical changes of premenstruum

    D. Awareness of general principles of vocal hygiene

    E. Identification of vocally abusive practices during premenstruum

    F. Elimination of vocally abusive practices

Contract Negotiation

Esther's level of commitment to improving her vocal behavior was so strong that the speech-language pathologist did not feel a contractual agreement was necessary. The decision was based on the fact that Esther was experiencing an acute, inconsistent pattern of symptoms rather than a chronic problem with severe symptomatology. Lifestyle factors are especially significant in such cases. If Esther had not been so involved with debating, she might not have noticed the intermittent changes in her vocal behavior.

The speech pathologist must be sensitive to the way in which an individual perceives and reacts to changes in voice. When reactions are intense and troublesome, they need to be addressed. Severity of symptoms, therefore, is not the only yardstick for defining a voice problem.

Therapy Plan

The consultation model seemed the most appropriate intervention strategy for Esther. Her high motivation and experience in researching topics for debate made her an excellent candidate for independent research and study on the topic of PMS and the voice. Esther met with the speech-language pathologist for 15-minute sessions during five study hall periods to learn about vocal hygiene. On each occasion, she received reading materials, assignments, and brief instruction. Since she was already evaluating her debate presentations on a tape recorder, this format for self-evaluation was continued.

Esther was so highly motivated that it was not necessary to develop programming to increase her internal motivation. Her problem was defined during discussions of vocal symptoms and during consultations with the medical specialist on PMS. Esther's voice program centered around analysis of the problem through knowledge acquisition and knowledge demonstration. As a result of her reading, Esther developed a list of PMS symptoms that specifically affected vocal interaction and a list of vocal hygiene rules for debaters.

◆ CARLOS: AN EXAMPLE OF MUTATIONAL FALSETTO

Carlos, age 17, was referred to the speech-language pathologist by his family doctor. He and his mother had consulted the physician concerning Carlos' high-pitched voice, which he found embarrassing. The medical report stated that Carlos was physically mature, there was no endocrine imbalance, and the laryngeal mechanism was within normal limits.

In the initial interview with the speech-language pathologist, Carlos appeared highly motivated and eager to pursue therapy. He stated that he had hoped that his voice would deepen as he grew older, but that didn't seem to be happening. He could produce a lower voice when he concentrated on it. However, when he was tense or excited, his pitch was extremely high and pitch breaks occurred frequently. He said this affected his social life since he avoided situations involving a lot of talking, and was especially shy when he was around girls.

The speech-language pathologist administered a pure tone hearing test and ascertained that Carlos' hearing was within normal limits bilaterally. The voice evaluation indicated that respiratory patterns for speech appeared to be within normal limits. Carlos spoke with reduced phonatory power at a habitually high pitch of approximately 163 Hz (with a conversational range of 132–177 Hz as measured on the Visi-Pitch) and used minimal pitch inflections; however, pitch breaks were noted when tension increased. At such times, phonation ceased temporarily and reappeared at a lower pitch level. When Carlos reacted negatively to these pitch breaks, his overall tension increased and his pitch resumed its higher level. He could produce loudness variations within normal limits during testing, although volume was habitually soft. Resonance patterns were appropriate, and no quality deviations were noted.

In discussions with Carlos, it emerged that he had a particularly close relationship with his mother, whom he perceived as supportive and understanding. He voiced some ambivalence regarding his relationship with his father, whom he admired for his professional success, but whose passion for hunting and aggressive activities were contrary to Carlos' more sensitive nature.

The speech-language pathologist hypothesized that Carlos may have been unable to habituate an adult male pitch because he was unconsciously equating it with those masculine qualities personified by his father, with whom he was unable to identify. The speech-language pathologist decided that voice therapy should include opportunities for Carlos to explore a variety of ways to express adult masculinity consistent with his own values and personality characteristics.

An outline and discussion of Carlos' voice therapy sequence follows.

Evaluation

  I. Factors Precipitating Negative Behaviors
    A. Psychosocial
      1. Equating adult male pitch level with personality characteristics personified by the father
      2. Lack of awareness of the range of acceptable adult masculine characteristics
  II. Negative Behaviors Observed
    A. Reduced loudness
    B. Limited inflection
    C. Immature pitch level
    D. Pitch breaks
    E. Anxiety reactions to pitch breaks
 III. Sample Target Behaviors for Therapy
    A. Analysis of relationship between pitch and perceptions of masculinity
    B. Lowered pitch level
    C. Increased use of inflectional patterns
    D. Increased loudness
    E. Reduction of anxiety in response to vocal behavior

Contract Negotiation

  I. Areas for Modification
    A. Phonation
    B. Respiration
    C. Interpersonal
  II. Ordering Targets
    A. Lowered pitch level
    B. Increased use of inflectional patterns
    C. Reduction of anxiety in response to vocal behavior
    D. Analysis of relationship between pitch and perceptions of masculinity
    E. Increased loudness

III. Matching Targets and Approaches
    A. Concurrent approach
    B. Acquisition of facts and information
       1. Readings
       2. Diagrams
       3. Discussions
       4. Instrumentation (Visi-Pitch, tuning fork, pitch pipe)
       5. Laryngeal model
       6. Written reports
       7. Observations
IV. Format for Implementation
    A. Frequency and length of contact with speech-language pathologist: twice per week for 45 minutes per session
    B. Type of contact: individual
    C. Non-credit (sessions scheduled during study hall)
    D. Speech-language pathologist's office
    E. Ninety percent attendance (not more than four absences)

Therapy Plan

Carlos was highly motivated and eager to pursue voice therapy because of embarrassment caused by his high vocal pitch. He was able to describe his problem and provide examples of how his voice limited his social interactions. Carlos was taught the relationships between air flow and vocal fold adjustments and the resulting pitch and loudness changes through the use of readings, diagrams, and models.

As an assignment Carlos read Dr. Morton Cooper's *Change Your Voice, Change Your Life* (1984), which provided an introduction to a general discussion of vocal and speaking styles. Although the speech-language pathologist felt that Carlos was confusing his stereotype of masculinity and his negative reactions to his father's speaking styles, the point was not addressed directly. Rather, the speech-language pathologist discussed how speakers sometimes cause listeners to react negatively because of sentence structure and tone of voice. Carlos listed the "hidden message" in statements such as:

◆ "I don't care how you feel about it, just do it." (*ordering*)
◆ "When I was your age..." (*preaching*)
◆ "You always look untidy. You kids are all alike." (*overgeneralizing*)
◆ "You probably feel that way because..." (*diagnosing*)

  I. Methods for Monitoring and Evaluating Progress
    A. Tuning fork (auditory)
    B. Visi-Pitch (visual)

    C. Logs

    D. Graphs

    E. Self-reports

    F. Video and audio tapes

II. Timelines for Treatment Schedule and Dismissal Criteria

    A. Level of proficiency to be achieved in each target area

        1. Lowered pitch level: habitual pitch level between 120–128 Hz (100 percent)

        2. Increased use of inflectional patterns: conversational range of 90–156 Hz (80 percent)

        3. Reduction of anxiety in response to vocal behavior (50 percent increase in self-reported initiation of social interactions)

        4. Analysis of relationship between pitch and perceptions of masculinity (B or above grade on written report summarizing data collected by personal observations)

        5. Increased loudness (demonstration of 90–100 dB level on (VU) meter, with microphone 2 inches from mouth, during 50-word reading passage

    B. Maximum duration of therapy: one semester

    C. Progress Review

        1. Dates for progress report: midsemester and end of semester

        2. Persons to receive progress report: physician, mother

        3. Date for termination, extension, or revision of treatment plan: end of each semester

    D. Frequency and type of follow-up after cessation of therapy sessions

        1. Frequency: once every other month for one semester

        2. Techniques: face-to-face or telephone interview

           a. self-evaluation

           b. evaluation of others

◆ ANNETTE: AN EXAMPLE OF REACTION TO EMOTIONAL TRAUMA

Annette, age 17, a senior in a large metropolitan high school, was referred to the speech-language pathologist by the music teacher, who was directing the annual school musical. The production was "Auntie Mame," and Annette was cast in the leading role.

The music teacher was concerned because of abrupt changes that had occurred in Annette's performance during rehearsals. He said that he had worked with Annette during previous productions with outstanding results, but that recently both her concentration and vocal skill had deteriorated markedly. He noted that her singing voice was characterized by restricted range and intermittent pitch breaks, she seemed unable to project her voice in speaking parts, and she seemed much less enthusiastic than in previous productions. He felt Annette was committed to the role, but her fears of "losing her high notes" and not being able to predict when her voice would break were reducing her overall confidence. He hoped that the speech-language pathologist could help Annette with her vocal problems, because he would have to recast the part if her performance did not improve significantly.

The speech-language pathologist had attended previous school musicals and had been impressed by Annette's strong vocal technique and vibrant stage personality. Since Annette's problems appeared to be related specifically to her on-stage vocal behavior, the speech-language pathologist decided to observe part of the next rehearsal period to see if the problem warranted intervention.

While watching part of the next rehearsal, the speech-language pathologist observed that Annette seemed generally subdued: her gestures and facial expressions were restricted, eye contact was poor, her voice was frequently inaudible, and pitch breaks occurred in the upper part of her singing range. She thought that Annette seemed depressed and withdrawn, but felt that short-term coaching on vocal projection techniques and eye contact awareness could improve Annette's performance.

The speech-language pathologist met with Annette and reviewed basic information concerning respiration and more precise articulation. Annette demonstrated that she understood the basic principles and was able to apply them during all of the exercises. She also demonstrated appropriate eye contact.

The speech-language pathologist decided that the difficulty must be related to Annette's inability to apply these principles while on-stage. She arranged for another member of the cast to meet with her and Annette in the auditorium. She wanted to see if Annette could transfer her fine performance in the speech room to the larger setting. Again, Annette's performance was flawless.

The speech-language pathologist believed that Annette's problem had been solved. However, two days later Annette reappeared in the speech-language pathologist's office in tears. She said that rehearsal the night before had been a disaster. She seemed utterly, despondent, and kept repeating, "I just can't go on with it!" She felt the only thing she could do was to withdraw from the production.

Lengthy discussion revealed that Annette froze on stage during every rehearsal because she was always aware that a member of the stage crew was staring at her from the wings. She said, "He watches me all the time, and I can't stand it! When I know he's there, I feel paralyzed." Amidst a flood of tears, Annette revealed that shortly after rehearsals for "Auntie Mame" began, she accepted a ride home from the young man. However, instead of driving her home, he had driven her to a secluded area and forcibly raped her. She was afraid to tell anyone about this since she felt it was her fault that she had unknowingly given him the impression that she was interested in him. She said he had told her it was her fault for leading him on. Although Annette felt she had treated him in the same manner as she had treated everyone else in the cast, she now questioned whether her outgoing personality could be misinterpreted. She had not told anyone about the incident because she wanted to forget it. She feared that her reputation would be ruined if anyone knew. However, she was filled with terror everytime she saw this boy.

The speech-language pathologist assured Annette that her feelings and reactions were typical of the reactions of the victims of rape. She said she could understand why Annette did not want others to know, but that she had done the correct thing by finally telling someone. The speech-language pathologist assured Annette that she understood the problems with rehearsals and advised Annette not to resign from the cast until they spoke again the next day.

An outline and discussion of Annette's voice therapy sequence follows.

Evaluation

I. Factors Precipitating Negative Behaviors
  A. Lifestyle
    1. Failure in situations that formerly held high value and reward
    2. Negative feedback from music director
    3. Demanding rehearsal schedule
  B. Interpersonal
    1. Rape by member of the stage crew
    2. Attempts to repress the traumatic event
    3. Fear that others may find out about the rape
    4. Guilt associated with her perception that she may have provoked the rape
II. Negative Behavior Observed
  A. Inability to perform on stage
    1. Poor eye contact
    2. Limited facial expression
    3. Restricted gestures

    4. Insufficient volume and breath support
    5. Inadequate oral movement
    6. Pitch breaks on high notes
    7. Limited pitch variation in speaking segments
III. Sample Target Behaviors for Therapy
    A. Awareness of typical reactions of rape victims
    B. Awareness of the need to inform and involve police/family
    C. Referral to support group for rape victims
    D. Awareness of relationship between emotional state and vocal behaviors
    E. Awareness of the need to consult with the music director
        1. Explanation of the problem
        2. Removal of rapist from the stage crew
        3. Referral of rapist for counseling
        4. Negotiations for mutual expectations regarding continued participation in the cast

Discussion

Although Annette's problem was not one the speech-language pathologist would normally be involved with, the fact that Annette had confided in her meant that the speech-language pathologist felt a responsibility to assist Annette in dealing with a very difficult situation. The speech-language pathologist realized that a case conference would have to be called as quickly as possible, but she also realized that she needed to talk more with Annette so that Annette would see the need to involve others. At their next meeting, the speech-language pathologist gave Annette readings to help her understand that her reactions were typical of others who had experienced similar trauma. Annette found *Top Secret* (see References) especially helpful. The speech-language pathologist also discussed some of the myths that exist about rape.

Following another meeting with the speech-language pathologist, Annette agreed to talk the problem over with her parents and asked that the speech-language pathologist talk to the music teacher and school principal. The parents, speech-language pathologist, music teacher, and principal discussed the management of the problem with an emphasis on the maintenance of confidentiality. Management strategies included:

♦ Referral to a community rape support group for ongoing counseling
♦ Medical evaluation by the family physician (because there is always the risk of internal injury, disease, or pregnancy)

- ♦ The principal agreed to assume responsibility for:
  1. Discussing the situation with both the boy and his parents
  2. Informing the boy and his parents that the police would be notified, and contacting the police
  3. Informing the boy that he was being removed from the production's stage crew and could not participate in or attend any segment of the production
  4. Investigating and recommending appropriate resources (e.g., counseling) to assist the boy
  5. Seeking reports and follow-up from counseling agencies
- ♦ The music teacher assumed responsibility for:
  1. Ensuring that the boy was not present at rehearsals or performances
  2. Monitoring Annette's vocal behavior and updating the speech-language pathologist
  3. Maintaining confidentiality concerning the problem with respect to the rest of the cast

The speech-language pathologist assumed responsibility for helping Annette become aware of the relationship between emotional state and vocal behavior and helping her practice techniques to reduce vocal tension. The speech-language pathologist and Annette agreed to meet once a week after school for 45 minutes. A six-week duration was agreed on.

The parents agreed to maintain contact with the music director, speech-language pathologist, and school principal as well as follow the suggestions of personnel in charge of the rape support group. They also volunteered to supervise car-pooling arrangements for Annette and her friends to and from extracurricular activities.

At adolescence, more than at any other life stage, new physical and psychosocial factors exert a profound influence on the individual. It is critical that all factors relevant to a voice problem be addressed. The case histories in this chapter illustrate a holistic approach to the modification of vocal symptoms which actively engages the students in the process of change.

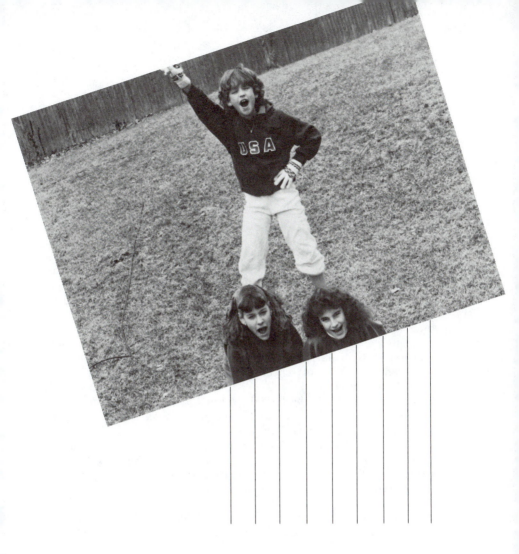

References and
Suggested Readings

Abritton, T. P. (1984, November). *Secondary speech-language programs: Strategies for a new delivery system.* Paper presented at the annual convention of the American-Speech-Language-Hearing Association, San Francisco.

Andrews, M. L. (1982). *Frequency characteristics of the voices of 740 Australian school children.* Unpublished manuscript, Indiana University, Bloomington, IN.

Andrews, M. L. (1986). *Voice therapy for children.* White Plaines, NY: Longman, Inc.

Andrews, M. L., & Shank, K. H. (1983). Some observations concerning the cheering behavior of school-girl cheerleaders. *Language, Speech, and Hearing Services in Schools, 14,* 150–156.

Aronson, A. E. (1973). *Psychogenic voice disorders: An interdisciplinary approach to detection, diagnosis and therapy: Audio seminars in speech pathology.* Philadelphia: Saunders.

Aronson, A. E. (1980). *Clinical voice disorders: An interdisciplinary approach.* New York: Brian C. Decker, a division of Thieme-Stratton, Inc.

Baken, R. J. (1979, June). Respiratory mechanisms: Introduction and overview. *Transcripts of the 8th Symposium: Care of the Professional Voice, 2,* 9–13.

Battle, D. W., & Van Hattum, R. J. (1982). Scheduling. In R. J. Van Hattum (Ed.), *Speech-language programming in the schools* (2nd ed., pp. 448–509). Springfield, IL: Thomas.

Bell, R. (1980). *Changing bodies, changing lives (A book for teens on sex and relationships).* New York: Random House.

Benson, H. (1975). *The relaxation response.* New York: Morrow.

Berryman, J. D. (1986). Clinical techniques and materials. In W. R. Neal (Ed.), *Speech-language pathology services in secondary schools* (pp. 99–122). Austin, TX: Pro-Ed.

Bless, D. M., & Abbs, J. H. (1983). *Vocal fold physiology: Contemporary research and clinical issues.* San Diego, CA: College-Hill Press.

Blos, P. (1962). *On adolescence.* New York: The Free Press.

Blyth, D. A., Simmons, R. G., & Carlton-Ford, S. (1983). The adjustment of early adolescents to school transitions. *Journal of Early Adolescence, 3*(1–2), 105–120.

Blyth, D. A., Thiel, K. S., Mitsch, D., & Simmons, R. G. (1980). Another look at school crime: Student as victim. *Youth and Society, 11*(3), 369–388.

Boone, D. R. (1974). Dismissal criteria in voice therapy. *Journal of Speech and Hearing Disorders, 39,* 133–139.

124

Boone, D. R. (1977). *The voice and voice therapy.* Englewood Cliffs, NJ: Prentice-Hall.

Boone, D. R. (1983). *The voice and voice therapy.* Englewood Cliffs, NJ: Prentice-Hall.

Bradford, M. A., Hosea, K. L., & Neal, W. R., Jr. (1977, November). *National survey of speech pathology services in the secondary schools.* Paper presented at the annual convention of the American Speech-Language-Hearing Association, Chicago.

Brammer, L. M. (1973). *The helping relationship process and skills.* Englewood Cliffs, NJ: Prentice-Hall.

Bramson, R., & Bramson, S. (1985). *The stressless home.* Garden City, NY: Anchor-Doubleday.

Brodnitz, F. S. (1963). Goals, results and limitations of vocal rehabilitation. *Archives of Otolaryngology, 77,* 148–156.

Brodnitz, F. S. (1971). *Vocal rehabilitation.* Rochester, MN: American Academy of Ophthamology and Otolaryngology.

Budoff, P. W. (1981). *No more menstrual cramps and other good news.* New York: Penguin Books.

Carkhuff, R. R. (1969). *Helping and human relations* (Vol. 2). New York: Holt, Rinehart & Winston.

Conger, J. J. (1973). *Adolescence and youth.* New York: Harper & Row.

Cooksey, J. M. (1977). The development of a contemporary eclectic theory for the training and cultivation of the junior high school male changing voice. *Music Educator's Journal, 10-12.*

Cooper, I. & Kuersteiner, K. O. (1970). *Teaching junior high school music* (2nd ed.). Boston: Allyn & Bacon.

Cooper, M. (1973). *Modern techniques of vocal rehabilitation.* Springfield, IL: Thomas.

Cooper, M. (1977). Direct vocal rehabilitation. In M. Cooper & M. H. Cooper (Eds.), *Approaches to vocal rehabilitation* (pp. 22–42). Springfield, IL: Thomas.

Cooper, M. (1984). *Change your voice, change your life.* New York: Noble Books.

Coopersmith, S. (1967). *The antecedents of self-esteem.* San Francisco: W. H. Freeman.

Dalton, K. (1977). *Premenstrual syndrome and progesterone therapy.* Chicago: Year Book.

Dalton, K. (1979). *Once a month.* Pomona, CA: Hunter House.

Dobson, J. (1984). *Preparing for adolescence.* New York: Bantam.

Douvan, E., & Adelson, J. (1966). *The adolescent experience.* New York: Wiley.

Eckel, F., & Boone, D. (1981). The s/z ratio as an indication of laryngeal pathology. *Journal of Speech and Hearing Disorders, 46,* 147–149.

Ekstrom, R. C. (1959). *Comparison of the male voice before, during and after mutation.* Doctoral dissertation, University of Southern California.

Espenschade, A. I., & Eckert, H. (1967). *Motor development.* Columbus, OH: Merrill.

Fay, J., & Flerchinger, B. J. (1982). *Top secret.* Renton, WA: King County Rape Relief.

Fellows, J. B. (1976). The speech pathologist in the high school setting. *Language, Speech and Hearing Services in Schools, 7*, 61–63.

Flach, M., Schwickardi, H., & Simon, R. (1969). What influence do menstruation and pregnancy have on the trained singing voice? *Folia Phoniatrica, 21*, 199–205.

Flynn, P. (1978). Effective clinical interviewing. *Language, Speech and Hearing Services in Schools, 9*, 265–271.

Fox, D. R. (1978). Evaluation of voice problems. In S. Singh & J. Lynch (Eds.), *Diagnostic procedures in hearing, language and speech* (pp. 485–527). Baltimore: University Park Press.

Frable, M. S. (1972). Hoarseness, a symptom of premenstrual tension. *Archives of Otolaryngology, 75*, 66–67.

Frassinelli, L., Superior, K., & Meyers, J. (1983). A consultation model for speech and language intervention. *Asha, 25*(11), 25–30.

Friesen, J. H. (1972). *Vocal mutation in the adolescent male: Its chronology and a comparison with fluctuations in musical interest.* DMA, University of Oregon.

Frisch, R. E. (1972). Weight at menarche: Similarity for well nourished and under-nourished girls at differing ages, and evidence for historical constancy. *Pediatrics, 50*, 445–450.

Frisch, R. E., & Revelle, R. (1970). Height and weight at menarche and a hypothesis of critical body weights and adolescent events. *Science, 169*, 397–399.

Frisch, R. E., & Revelle, R. (1971a). Height and weight of girls and boys at the time of initiation of the adolescent growth spurt in height and weight and the relationship to menarche. *Human Biology, 43*, 140–159.

Frisch, R. E., & Revelle, R. (1971b). Height and weight at menarche and a hypothesis of menarche. *Archives of Disease in Children, 46*, 695–701.

Frisch, R. E., Revelle, R., & Cook, S. (1973). Components of the critical weight at menarche and at initiation of the adolescent growth spurt: Estimated total water, lean body mass and fat. *Human Biology, 45*, 469–483.

Goda, S. (1970). *Articulation therapy and consonant drillbook.* New York: Grune & Stratton.

Greene, M. C. L. (1972). *The voice and its disorders* (3rd ed.). New York: Pitman.

Gregory, H. H. (1986). The clinician's attitudes. In *Counseling Stutterers* (No. 18, pp. 9–17). Memphis, TN: Speech Foundation of America.

Grinder, R. E. (1973). *Adolescence.* New York: Wiley.

Hamachek, D. E. (1978). *Encounters with the self* (2nd ed). New York: Holt, Rinehart & Winston.

Handler, S. D., & Witmore, R. (1982). Otolaryngologic injuries. *Clinical Sports Medicine, 1*, 431–447.

Hanley, T. D., & Thurman, W. L. (1970). *Developing vocal skills* (2nd ed.). New York: Holt, Rinehart & Winston.

Harrison, M. (1982). *Self-help for premenstrual syndrome.* Cambridge, MA: Matrix Press.

Hately, B. W., Evison, G., & Samuel, E. (1965). The pattern of ossification in the laryneal cartilages: A radiological study. *British Journal of Radiology, 38*, 585–591.

Helmi, A. M., El-Ghazzawi, I. F., Mandour, M., & Shehata, M. A. (1975). The effect of oestrogen on the nasal respiratory mucosa. *Journal of Laryngology and Otology, 89*(12), 1229–1241.

Hirano, M. (1974). Morphological structure of the vocal cord as a vibrator and its variations. *Folia Phoniatrica, 26,* 89–94.

Hirano, M. (1981). Structure of the vocal fold in normal and disease states. *American Speech and Hearing Association Reports 11,* Rockville, MD.

Hirano, M., Kurita, S., & Nasashima, T. (1981). The structure of the vocal folds. In *Vocal fold physiology* (pp. 33–44). Tokyo: University of Tokyo Press.

Hollien, H., & Malcik, E. (1962, March). Adolescent voice changes in southern negro males. *Speech Monographs, 29,* 53–58.

Hollien, H., & Malcik, E. (1967). Evaluation of cross-sectional studies of adolescent voice change in males. *Speech Monographs, 34,* 80–84.

Hollien, H., Malcik, E., & Hollien, B. (1965). Adolescent voice changes in southern white males. *Speech Monographs, 32,* 87–90.

Jensen, P. (1964). Hoarseness in cheerleaders. *Asha, 6,* 406.

Jerome, J. (1980). *The sweet spot in time.* New York: Summit Books, pp. 242–264.

Jones, D., Austin, C., MacLean, D., & Warkomski, R. (1973). Task force report on traditional scheduling procedures in schools. *Language, Speech, and Hearing Services in Schools, 4,* 100–109.

Jones, M. C. (1958). A study of socialization patterns at the high school level. *Journal of Genetic Psychology, 93,* 87–111.

Jones, M. C. (1965). Psychological correlates of somatic development. *Child Development, 36,* 899–911.

Jones, M. C., & Bayley, N. (1950). Physical maturing among boys as related to behavior. *Journal of Educational Psychology, 41,* 129–148.

Jones, M. C., & Mussen, P. H. (1958). Self-conceptions, motivations, and interpersonal attitudes of early and late maturing girls. *Child Development, 29,* 491–501.

Jones, M. M. (1983, August). Premenstrual syndrome: Part 1. *British Journal of Sexual Medicine, 10*(99), 9–11.

Joseph, L., & Mills, A. (1983). *A doctor discusses allergy: Fact and fiction.* Chicago: Budlong.

Joseph, W. (1963, Summer). Vocal growth in the human adolescent and the total growth process. *Journal of Music Education, 13,* 135.

Josselyn, I. M. (1962). *The adolescent and his world.* New York: Family Service Association of America.

Judson, L. S. V., & Weaver, A. T. (1965). *Voice science* (2nd ed.). New York: Appleton-Century-Crofts.

Kagan, Jerome (1971, Fall). A conception of early adolescence. *Daedalus, 100*(4), 997–1012.

Kahane, J. C. (1978). A morphological study of the human prepubertal and pubertal larynx. *American Journal of Anatomy, 151,* 11–20.

Kahane, J. C. (1980). Age related histological changes in the human male and female laryngeal cartilages: Biological and functional implications. In V. Lawrence (Ed.), *Transcripts of the Ninth Symposium: Care of the Professional Voice, Part I* (pp. 11–20). New York: The Voice Foundation.

Kahane, J. C. (1982). Growth and development of the human prepubertal and pubertal larynx. *Journal of Speech and Hearing Research, 25,* 446–455.

Kahane, J. C. (1983). Age related changes in the elastic fibres of the adult male vocal ligament. In V. Lawrence (Ed.), *Transcripts of the Eleventh Symposium: Care of the Professional Voice.* New York: The Voice Foundation.

Kahane, J. C. (1983, August). Postnatal development and aging of the human larynx. *Seminars in Speech and Language, 4*(3), 189–203.

Kanter, R. M. (1983). *The change masters.* London: Counterpoint, Unwin Paperbacks.

Kiell, N. (1964). *The universal experience of adolescence.* Boston: Beacon Press.

Klock, L. E., Jr. (1968). *The growth and development of the human larynx from birth to adolescence.* Unpublished master's thesis, University of Washington School of Medicine, Seattle.

Knorr, D., Bidlingmaier, O., Butenandt, H. F., & Ehrt-Wehle, R. (1974). Plasma testosterone in male puberty. *Acta Endocrinologia, 75,* 181–194.

Kohlberg, L. (1975). Moral development in the schools: A developmental view. In R. E. Grinder (Ed.), *Studies in adolescence* (3rd ed.). New York: Macmillan.

Kronberg, J., Tyano, S., Apter, A., & Wijsenbeck, H. (1981). Treatment of transsexualism in adolescence. *Journal of Adolescence, 4,* 177–185.

Kubler-Ross, E. (1969). *On death and dying.* New York: Macmillan.

Kulin, H. E., Grumbach, M. M., & Kaplan, S. L. (1972). Gonadal-hypothalamic interaction in prepubertal and pubertal man: Effect of clomisphene citrate on urinary follicle-stimulating hormone and luteinizing hormone and plasma testosterone. *Pediatric Research, 6,* 162–171.

Large, J., & Patton, R. (1979, June). The effects of weight training and aerobic exercise on singers. *Transcripts of the Eighth Symposium: Care of the Professional Voice, 1,* 29–35.

Laughlin, H. P. (1970). *The ego and its defences.* New York: Appleton-Century-Crofts.

Laver, J. (1980). *The phonetic descripton of voice quality.* New York: Cambridge University Press.

Lehiste, I. (1976). Suprasegmental features of speech. In N. J. Lass (Ed.), *Contemporary issues in experimental phonetics.* New York: Academic Press.

Lerman, J. W., & Damste, P. H. (1969). Voice pitch of homosexuals. *Folia Phoniatrica, 21*(5), 340–346.

Luchsinger, R, & Arnold, G. E. (1965). *Voice-speech-language clinical communicology: Its physiology and pathology.* Belmont, CA: Wadsworth.

Maccoby, E., & Jacklin, C. N. (1974). *The psychology of sex differences.* Stanford, CA: Stanford University Press.

Marshall, W. A., & Tanner, J. M. (1969). Variations in pattern of pubertal changes in girls. *Archives of Disease in Children, 45,* 291–303.

Marshall, W. A., & Tanner, J. M. (1970). Variations in the patterns of pubertal changes in boys. *Archives of Disease in Childhood, 45,* 13–23.

McCandless, B. R., & Coop, R. H. (1979). *Adolescents: Behavior and development* (2nd ed.). New York: Holt, Rinehart & Winston.

McGlone, R. E., & Hollien, H. (1963). Vocal pitch characteristics of aged women. *Journal of Speech and Hearing Research, 6,* 164–167.

McKenzie, D. (1956). *Training the boy's changing voice.* New Brunswick, NJ: Rutgers University Press.

McKinley, N. L., & Lord-Larsen, V. (1985). Neglected language-disordered adolescent: A delivery model. *Language, Speech and Hearing Services in Schools, 16,* 2–15.

Miller, D. (1974). *Adolescence: Psychology, psychopathology and psychotherapy.* New York: Jason Aronson.

Mischel, W. (1970). Sex-typing and socialization. In P. H. Mussen (Ed.), *Carmichael's manual of child psychology* (Vol. 2, 3rd ed., pp. 3–72). New York: John Wiley.

Money, J., & Clopper, R. R., Jr. (1974, February). Psychosocial and psychosexual aspects of errors of prepubertal onset and development. *Human Biology, 46*(1), 173–181.

Morris, H. L., Spriesterbach, D. C., & Darley, F. L. (1961). An articulation test for assessing competency of velopharyngeal closure. *Journal of Speech and Hearing Research, 4,* 48–55.

Mussen, P. H., & Jones, M. C. (1957). Self-conceptions, motivations and interpersonal attitudes of late- and early-maturing boys. *Child Development, 28,* 243–256.

Muuss, R. E. (1975). *Theories of adolescence* (3rd ed.). New York: Random House.

Naidr, J., Zboril, M., & Ševčik, K. (1965). Die pubertalen veränderungen der stimme bie junger im verlauf von 5 jahren. *Folia Phoniatrica, 17:* 1–18.

Neal, W. R., Jr. (1976). Speech pathology services in secondary schools. *Language, Speech and Hearing Services in Schools, 7,* 6–16.

Neal, W. R., Jr. (1986). *Speech-language pathology services in secondary schools.* Austin, TX: Pro-Ed.

Neidecker, R. A. (1980). *School progress in speech-language: Organization and management.* Englewood Cliffs, NJ: Prentice-Hall.

Osterrieth, P. A. (1969). Adolescence: Some psychological aspects. In G. Caplan & S. Lebovici (Eds.), *Adolescence: Psychosocial perspectives* (pp. 11–21). New York: Basu Books.

O'Toole, T. J., & Zaslow, E. L. (1969). Public school speech and hearing programs: Things are changing. *Asha, 11,* 499–501.

Pannbacker, M. (1984). Classification systems of voice disorders: A review of the literature. *Language, Speech and Hearing Services in Schools, 15*(3), 169–174.

Pasquariello, P. S., Potsic, W. P., Miller, L., & Corso, C. (1983). Nutrition in adenotonsillar hyperplasia. Paper presented at the annual meeting of SENTAC, San Diego, CA.

Pedry, C. P. (1945). A study of voice change in boys between the ages of eleven and sixteen. *Speech Monographs, 12,* 30–36.

Perkins, W. H. (1977). *Speech pathology: An applied behaviral science* (2nd ed.). St. Louis: C. V. Mosby.

Piaget, J. (1974). Adolescence: Thought and its operation: The affectivity of the personality in the social world of adults. In Z. M. Cantwell & P. N.

Svajian (Eds.), *Adolescence: Studies in development.* (pp. 34–56). Itasco, IL: Peacock.

Prange, A. (1974). *The thyroid axis, drugs and behavior.* New York: Raven Press.

Prater, R. J., & Swift, R. W. (1984). *Manual of voice therapy.* Boston: Little, Brown.

Ptacek, P. H., & Sander, E. K. (1963). Maximum duration of phonation. *Journal of Speech and Hearing Disorders, 28,* 171.

Punt, N. (1983). Laryngology applied to singers and actors. *Journal of Laryngology and Otology* (Suppl. 6), 1–24.

Punt, N. A. (1979). *Singer's and actor's throat* (3rd ed.). New York: Drama Book Specialists.

Randolph, T., & Moss, R. (1981). *An alternative approach to allergies.* New York: Lippincott & Crowell.

Reich, A., McHenry, M., & Keaton, A. (1986). A survey of dysphonic episodes in high school cheerleaders. *Language, Speech and Hearing Services in Schools, 17*(1), 63–71.

Reiter, E. O. (1981, January). Delayed puberty in boys. *Medical Aspects of Human Sexuality, 15*(1), 79–80.

Rogers, C. R. (1961). *On becoming a person.* Boston: Houghton-Mifflin.

Sadewitz, V. L., & Shprintzen, R. J. (1985, December). *Changes in velopharyngeal closure with age.* Paper presented at the annual meeting of SENTAC, Dallas.

Sataloff, R. T. (1981, August). Professional singers: The science and art of clinical care. *American Journal of .Otolaryngology, 2*(3), 251–266.

Silverman, E. M., & Zimmer, C. (1978). Effect of the menstrual cycle on voice quality. *Archives of Otolaryngology, 104,* 7–10.

Smith-Frable, M. A. (1961). Hoarseness, a symptom of premenstrual tension. *Archives of Otolaryngology, 75,* 66–68.

Specter, P., Subtelny, J. D., Whitehead, R. L., & Wirz, S. L. (1979). Description and evaluation of a training program designed to reduce vocal tension in adult deaf speakers. *Volta Review, 81*(2).

Stathopoulos, E. T., & Weismer, G. (1985). Oral air flow and intraoral air pressure: A comparative study of children, youths and adults. *Folia Phoniatrica, 37,* 152–159.

Swanson, F. J. (1960). Music teaching in the junior high and school music. *Music Education Journal, 46*(4), 50.

Tait, N. A., Michel, J. P., & Carpenter, M. A. (1980). Maximum duration of sustained /s/ and /z/ in children. *Journal of Speech and Hearing Disorders, 45,* 239.

Tanner, J. M. (1971). Sequence, tempo, and individual variation in the growth and development of boys and girls aged twelve to sixteen. *Daedalus, 100,* 907–930.

Thomas, J. K. (1973). Adolescent endocrinology for counsellors of adolescents. *Adolescence, 8*(31), 395–406.

Todd, T. (1983, August). The steroid predicament. *Sports Illustrated, 59,* 62–72.

Toppozada, H., Michaels, L., Toppozada, M., El Ghazzawi, E., Talaat, A., & Elwany, S. (1981, December). The human nasal mucosa in the menstrual cycle. *Journal of Laryngology and Otology, 95,* 1237–1247.

Tosi, O., Postan, D., & Bianculli, C. (1976). Longitudinal study of children's voices at puberty. In E. Lorbell (Ed.), *Proceedings of the XVIth International Congress on Logopedics and Phoniatrics* (pp. 486–490). Basel: Karger.

Truax, C. B., & Carkhuff, R. R. (1967). *Toward effective counseling and psychotherapy.* Chicago: Aldine.

Van Gelder, L. (1974). Psychosomatic aspects of endocrine disorders of the voice. *Journal of Communication Disorders, 7,* 263–267.

Van Hattum, R. (1969). Program scheduling. In R. J. Van Hattum (Ed.), *Clinical speech in schools: Organization and management* (pp. 163–195). Springfield, IL: Thomas.

Wegscheider-Gruse, S. (1983). *Choice making for codependents, adult children and spirituality seekers.* Pompano Beach, FL: Health Communications.

Weiss, D. A. (1950). The pubertal chang of the human voice. *Folia Phoniatrica, 2*(3), 30–32.

Wilson, D. K. (1979). *Voice problems of children* (2nd ed.). Baltimore: Williams & Wilkins.

Wilson, D. K. (1987). *Voice problems of children* (3rd ed.). Baltimore: Williams & Wilkins.

Winder, A. E. (1974). Normal adolescence: Psychological factors. In A. E. Winder (Ed.), *Adolescence: Contemporary studies* (2nd ed.). New York: Van Nostrand.

Zemlin, W. R. (1968). *Speech and hearing science, anatomy and physiology.* Englewood Cliffs, NJ: Prentice-Hall.

Zemlin, W. R. (1981). *Speech and hearing science* (2nd ed.). Englewood Cliffs, NJ: Prentice-Hall.

Zehr, A. (1983). Beating the blues. *Potentials in human development (pp. 1–4).* Bloomington, IN: South Central Community Mental Health Center.

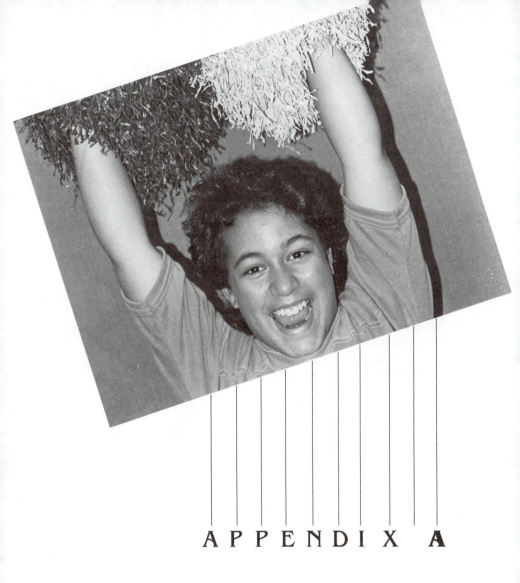

APPENDIX **A**

Practice Materials for Voice Therapy

In the following appendices, specific examples of practice materials for awareness, facilitating production, easy vocal production, and complex vocal production are presented. These activities can be used with a variety of voice disorders.

♦ CONTENTS

♦ *FACILITATORS*

Facilitators are used to stimulate an appropriate phonational pattern and are cues that are eliminated as the desired behavior stabilizes.

To Increase Laryngeal Tension
(useful when vocal fold closure needs strengthening)

1. Push/press while phonating
   a. push against a wall with two hands
   b. push a chair across the room
   c. push clasped hands together
   d. push hands down on seat of chair (while seated)
   e. push feet firmly against floor
   f. push clasped hands together behind body (this keeps shoulders back and enhances breathing)
   g. push hands against a table edge while seated

2. Pull while phonating
   a. pull on own fingers
   b. pull on a cord held by clinician
   c. pull on a lock of hair
   d. pull on a ledge or table edge

3. Sudden body movements while phonating
   a. thrust arm (with clenched fist) forward from chest position to full extension in front of chest
   b. kick leg forward (as in a chorus line kick)
   c. quick deep knee bends
   d. quick side bends (arm moves down outer leg)
   e. partial sit-ups
   f. "reach for the sky"

4. Visualization while phonating
   a. squeezed or constricted images (e.g., necktie too tight)
   b. frightening situations (e.g., standing on the edge of a cliff and loosing balance)
   c. strong emotional states (e.g., shrieks, cries, closed vowels, clenched jaw)

To Decrease Laryngeal Tension
(useful when folds are adducted with too much tension)

1. Vegetative movements while phonating
   a. chewing
   b. sighing
   c. yawning
   d. panting
   e. whistling

2. Body movements while phonating
   a. head rolls
   b. shoulder shrugs and rolls (can be done in unison and alternately)
   c. flop over at waist (Raggedy Anne style)
   d. lie flat on floor or table
   e. relaxed deep breathing
   f. twist back and forth from the torso

3. Speech movements
   a. drop jaw (to release tension in suprahyoids)
   b. blow out on voiceless continuants in a relaxed manner
   c. blow out on "whoo"
   d. hum to relaxing music
   e. intersperse "hums" with "h" in a relaxed sequence
   f. let voice flow through an open throat as "flow" is prolonged
   g. contrast very tense "i" with an open relaxed "a"

4. Images/visualization while phonating
   a. float on water while saying "hmm"
   b. feel "fat cheeks" like chipmunk while saying "aah"
   c. sink onto a soft feather bed while saying "oh"
   d. recapture own most relaxed situation or image
   e. drop word "blop" into a deep well (gradually increase number of "blops")
   f. think of honey or velvet (or other substance) and say "soothing"
   g. pretend to be quieting an agitated child/animal and murmur "There, there"
   h. visualize and adopt a relaxed posture; align head and torso and stand tall

To Increase Forward Placement of Voice
(useful to improve oral resonance)

1. Body position while phonating
   a. bend over from waist and feel voice falling forward toward floor
   b. place chin on folded arms on a table (while seated) and feel facial bones vibrating
   c. place hands on face and feel vibration
   d. push hands against sternum with an upward movement
   e. cup hands on either side of mouth, feel mouth opening, and project

2. Tactile cues while phonating
   a. hum and make the lips tickle
   b. practice frontal voiced plosives with vowels and "throw" the voice past the plosive (CVs)
   c. sing a song to "la," emphasizing tongue movement and mouth opening
   d. use the lips to push the voice forward
   e. "bite off" each word with precise articulation
   f. feel as if mouth opening and lip and tongue movements are exaggerated; watch in a mirror to check perceptions

3. Visualization while phonating
   a. pull an imaginary string of voice from the mouth
   b. "throw" the voice to a distant surface, listener, object
   c. pretend to have a hinged jaw and open it wide like a ventriloquist's dummy
   d. pretend to be an authority figure and speak with a declamatory vocal style
   e. pretend to be angry and "hit" the listener with each firmly articulated word

♦ *PRACTICE MATERIALS WITHOUT NASAL SOUNDS*

Words With Voiced Continuant Consonants

These words are suitable for improving oral resonance. Initially, words can be read in a "chanting" style, prolonging the vowels and voiced consonants. When appropriate oral resonance has been achieved, the words should be read in a conversational style, maximizing the consonants as "sound carriers." Care should be taken to avoid devoicing continuant consonants in final positions.

Monosyllabic		Multisyllabic	
rye	woe	rely	arouse
wave	woo	visa	rally
there	raise	Zulu	lazy
ooze	eyes	yellow	viral
live	ray	vowel	viva
rail	loaves	valley	volley
wise	raves	value	layers
use	zoo	vary	ravel
views	eve	very	losers
lull	wool	lathers	always
these	lathes	lazily	razor
owes	rouge	treasure	levers
veil	will	weasel	rather
vial	lose	lilly	lovely
zeal	veal	rosy	easily
czar	valve	revel	Lizzie
awes	low	Loyola	every
laws	zee	zero	early
Liz	zoe	rosary	leveler
rose	ewes	revise	livelier
whiz	lies	Eloise	easel
the	owes	they'll	zither
thou	wheeze	although	Louisa
thy	wise	leather	whereas
writhes	they	weather	realize
lair	though	worthy	they've
Lou	loathe	Larry	either
ale	wreathes	worthily	whithers
oil	Lear	Laura	worrier
raw	liar	Leah	larvae
row	eel	leeway	lava
rouse	zeal	really	layer
wave	real	olive	leery
wall	reels	oily	leisure
weave	rise	velour	resolve
all	rolls	evolve	valves
weigh	rules	revolve	elves

Words Without Nasal Consonants

The plosive and fricatives should be produced with emphasis on mouth opening and articulatory precision. These words are useful for students who need to experience "orality" and concentrate on continuity of velopharyngeal closure to generate appropriate oral pressure. Sentences to practice production of pressure consonants may also be used, such as, "These chillies are cheaper but these chips of Charlie's are best" and "Space visitors are cheapskate shoppers who are churlish to shopkeepers."

Monosyllabic		Multisyllabic	
take	weld	police	broccoli
clock	scold	bracelet	jeweled
beach	gauze	luggage	outrigger
coat	bat	breakfast	tablecloth
dart	cut	attractive	spaghetti
sport	dot	delicious	factory
book	feet	parachute	distributor
glue	hut	vegetable	duplicator
hook	put	selective	hospital
five	pit	shapeless	operator
puff	tot	tadpole	diversity
tip	let	helicopter	favorable
dead	rat	freaky	behavior
hit	root	disbelief	fertilizer
pill	spit	relative	vaporizer
cave	bite	variety	pleasure
kite	bath	perspire	precipice
fuzz	door	powerful	precocious
wag	deer	isolated	rebellious
bug	house	reflective	ridiculous
shout	row	celebrate	phosphorus
touch	food	bicycle	addressed
tell	hook	practical	righteous
light	bait	jealous	accessory
brow	good	pretzel	asphalt
cold	cash	shoelace	scoreboard
fruit	couch	cockroach	stethoscope
street	race	witchcraft	wastebasket
chop	sail	sauerkraut	escalator
rush	shake	chapter	discouraged
huge	chair	acrobatics	exposure
bulge	chill	chocolate	exchequer
golf	verb	irradiate	luxurious
fresh	loaf	refrigerate	paperbacks

(continued)

Words Without Nasal Consonants *(continued)*

Monosyllabic		Multisyllabic	
tweed	haul	jubilee	preserved
froze	yield	valuable	biweekly
doubt	child	exclusive	backlash
drool	vase	exclude	heckler

Sentences Without Nasal Consonants

1. I will purchase the vegetables for supper.
2. Bagels are Phillip's favorite food.
3. You are requested to stay here, Patricia.
4. Steve works at a very large store.
5. The subway fire caused great fright.
6. Jack always washes his face with soap.
7. Where do you wish to go?
8. He shouted loudly to the lady across the street.
9. The holidays passed altogether too quickly.
10. The picture of you is absolutely beautiful.
11. Who will give us the gist of this topic?
12. What vegetables would you like to have at the party?
13. She had to go back to school.
14. How do you like your eggs cooked?
15. I saw her go out to greet Peter.
16. Yesterday she wore a bright red suit with white shoes.
17. The celebrity was happy to receive the key to the city.
18. The girl was a popular Ohio State cheerleader.
19. The letter gave her a severe shock.
20. Food is so costly these days that it costs us $60 for a week's groceries.
21. He will be grateful to you for it.
22. There was too little variety of topics listed.
23. I had the watch repaired at the local jewelers.
24. The crawl stroke is easy to do.
25. This toothpaste is available at all reputable drug stores.
26. Tell her to be sure to address the parcels correctly.
27. The effects of alcohol are quite disastrous for drivers.
28. The college is situated here.
29. There will be a large art display at the state gallery this week.
30. The sailors had good weather throughout their voyage.
31. We have to stay at the library to study effectively.
32. Is she very seriously hurt?
33. I'd like a table for two over by the fireplace.
34. The subdued lights threw weird shadows about the hall.
35. I would like to travel overseas this year.
36. Basketball develops athletic skill.
37. The gatekeeper told the picketers to go away.
38. Will you give this boy a piece of paper?
39. I walked up the stairway before he did.
40. At sea the air is oppressively sultry.
41. We took the videotape to the class party.
42. Read your words aloud to the class.
43. Look before you leap or you'll fall up the stairs.
44. Good posture is a requisite to good speech.
45. The political party usually forgets its earlier pledges.
46. The library clerk is very polite.
47. Yes, I shall wait here for you.

Paragraphs Without Nasal Sounds

Our resort offers exotic local food that tastes as good as it looks. Beautiful, fresh, delicious appetizers to desserts are offered here. Fruits, vegetables, cakes, plus pies are all available for you. There are lots of places to go. These trips take you everywhere. Places such as Europe, Israel plus Florida. There is lots to do at these resorts. Your are able to sail, water ski, scuba dive, horseback ride, or sit at the pool. You will see lots of people at the resort; the guests plus workers will help you feel relaxed as well as happy.

Everybody loves to eat pizza. There are several foods that are good with which to top a pizza. Cheese is the best, but I also like sausage. Chili peppers are delicious, too. Olives are also OK. If I go to the pizzeria, I also order garlic bread. Plus, I'll get a salad. Rarely do I order all three together, though. I'd be obese if I did. As it is I eat a lot of pizza, so I usually have to watch what I eat. If I eat pizza everyday, I'll look like a hippo.

Just outside of Chicago there's a little old village called Libertyville. It is a beautiful area filled with history. A circle of large rose bushes that flatters the aged village hall borders the village square. Daily visitors cheerfully gaze at the colorful roses. The village square is a place for local artists or actors. People love to watch or participate with these activities while the sky is bright above. After the dark sky has appeared, refreshed visitors stroll by the lake that glows like a colorful glass. Few people realize Libertyville has this delightful character.

Charles just switched jobs. Because his wife, Debbie, works, too, they have extra cash to pay for a house. They hope to locate a big yellow house with a large yard that's close to the busy city. They chose the colors for the various places — lots of blues or reds. They have already picked out the chairs, tables, pillows plus little objects with which to decorate. They're really excited to look for a house especially because they expect their first baby after a short while.

There are very few areas of life that allow us to regard this world without disgust, but there is a beauty that people create out of the chaos: the pictures they produce, the lyrics they create, the books they write, plus the lives they lead. Of all these, the richest beauty is a life well lived. That is the perfect work of art.

Koala bears look like large, gray teddy bears. They are two to three feet tall with thick woolly fur. Trees serve as the chief habitat for koalas, especially eucalyptus trees. The foliage of the eucalyptus, as well as a few other trees, provides food for the creatures. Koalas occupy various parts of Australia. There is a risk that the species will disappear as eucalyptus trees are destroyed. To forestall this, koalas are protected by law.

Here are a few tips for the racquetball player. First, buy a good quality glove. Good sturdy plastic glasses are also a good idea to protect your eyes. You will also have to buy two racquetballs. After you have bought all the prerequisite articles, you are ready to play. Always be sure to keep the face of the racquet parallel to the wall you wish to hit. Last, try to hit the ball as close to the floor as possible.

Oral/Nasal Contrast Words

/m/	/b/	/m/	/b/
me	be	bomb	Bob
mail	bail	boom	boob
mar	bar	bum	bub
mass	bass	came	Cabe
mess	Bess	come	cub
my	bye	cram	crab
mill	Bill	dam	dab
mole	bowl	dim	dib
moss	boss	dumb	dub
muff	buff	limb	lib
mug	bug	loam	lobe
male	bail	game	Gabe
moan	bone	gram	grab
mow	bow	rim	rib
mile	bile	Jim	jib

/n/	/d/	/n/	/d/
gnome	dome	an	add
knave	Dave	ban	bad
knead	deed	been	bead
new	dew	Ben	bed
knock	dock	bin	bid
know	dough	bone	bode
Nan	Dan	bun	Budd
near	dear	clan	clad
neck	deck	clown	cloud
nice	dice	cone	code
Nile	dial	crown	crowd
nip	dip	dune	dude
nun	done	green	greed
nor	door	hen	head
nose	doze	Jane	jade
knot	dot	June	Jude
noun	down	lane	laid
numb	dumb	lean	lead
neigh	day	moon	mood
Newell	dual	prune	prude
name	dame	gone	God
note	dote	brawn	broad

(continued)

Oral/Nasal Contrast Words *(continued)*

/ŋ/	/g/	/ŋ/	/g/
bang	bag	lung	lug
bing	big	ping	pig
bong	bog	rang	rag
bring	brig	ring	rig
ding	dig	rung	rug
dong	dog	sang	sag
dung	dug	slang	slag
fang	fag	spring	sprig
gang	gag	swing	swig
hang	hag	tongue	tug
hung	hug	wing	wig
long	log	tang	tag

◆ *PRACTICE MATERIALS WITH NASAL SOUNDS*

Words With Nasal Consonants

Monosyllabic (vowels and voiced continuants only)		Monosyllabic (other consonants)	
name	male	mange	march
ming	mall	mink	mask
mane	nine	mound	mat
man	ring	monk	mace
mean	knees	mind	mash
numb	nouns	mumps	math
moan	mourn	manned	mass
moon	gnarl	mount	month
none	noun	malt	ninth
mine	gnaw	map	nip
gnome	known	nod	nix
noon	men	north	nook
norm	maim	not	neat
mine	ma'am	nest	next
mum	nun	knife	gnats
maize	noise	gnash	nights

Multisyllabic (vowels and voiced continuants only)		Multisyllabic (other consonants)	
aiming	mammogram	neutron	Cincinnati
morning	aluminum	amend	snakeskin
meaning	neon	nomad	centennial
Maureen	immune	mandate	monkey
family room	mammal	maintain	humdrum
linoleum	numbing	member	income
neoplasm	minimum	mental	nimble
enamel	membrane	milky	mushroom
mingle	hangman	minstrel	phantom
newsmen	Miami	mountain	springtime
ringing	normal	madam	symptom
anagram	animal	moonbeam	addendum
dining room	noisy	phoneme	pantomime
nasals	Norman	random	chrysanthemum
northern	neither	sternum	almond
naval	nylon	tandem	compendium

(continued)

Words With Nasal Consonants (continued)

Multisyllabic (vowels and voiced continuants only)	Multisyllabic (other consonants)	
pneumonia	anteroom	Hinduism
nominee	antonym	cannibalism
nouveau	Christendom	crematorium
lunar	maximum	abnormal
manner	synonym	informal
money	journalism	monument
owner	mongolism	ornament
inner	Anglicanism	number
airliner	condominium	magnificent
another	subnormal	coming
honors	almanac	England
lanolin	Monday	metholatum
lawn mower	lenient	international
maneuver	November	Pan-American
Manila	nonentity	nuisance
vanilla	ping pong	semifinal
mariner	gangplank	newborn
manually	Michigan	symposium
minerals	moment	nutmeg

Names With Nasal Consonants

Ways to use name lists include (1) reading all names of people you know, (2) reading all names containing more than one nasal sound, (3) reading all names that can be either a first or last name, (4) making up surnames containing nasal sounds, to go with the first names, (5) making up nicknames for as many of the names on the list as possible.

Mame	Mable	Moya	Murray
Maureen	Maurice	Mickie	Myrna
Marc	Marcus	Millie	Myron
May	Marie	Milton	Myrtle
Marvin	Marshall	Mandy	McArthur
Michael	Marsha	Mitchell	McIntosh
Matthew	Martin	Molly	Madeline
Myles	Mary	Morris	Madonna
Manuel	Mercedes	Meredith	Miranda
Amy	Emma	Jimmy	Jamie
Mimi	Omar	Remus	Sammy
Simon	Tammy	Timothy	Tommy
Kenneth	Edmond	Clementine	Pamela
Kimberly	Naomi	Adam	Christine
Alma	Elmer	Wilma	Thelma
Selma	Selina	Andrew	Edna
Nancy	Erma	Norma	Charmaine
Angela	Nanette	Smith	Neil
Nell	Nicholas	Nelson	Noel
Nina	Natalie	Napoleon	Anna
Annette	Lena	Benjamin	Bonny
Daniel	Dennis	Frances	Gina
Janet	Jeanette	Lana	Penelope
Venus	Robin	Mona	Blaine
Glenn	Donald	Dean	Jean
John	Joan	Lynn	Ronald
Stan	Shawn	Shane	Elaine
Eugene	Gordon	Helen	Herman
Irene	Karen	Susan	Colleen
Clinton	Aileen	Lyndon	Loraine
Sharon	Sanford	Sheldon	Sylvan
Allison	Sandra	Geraldine	Josephine
Shirleen	Magdalene	Vernon	Janice
Brandy	Cynthia	Indira	Blondie
Roland	Mary Ann	Ingrid	Bernard
Arnold	Ernest	Lorna	Lillian
Lorne	Spencer	Penny	Garland

Sentences With Nasal Consonants

1. No one knows Norman's nickname.
2. The Indians camped around the mountain.
3. Ken wants to go to Sweden next autumn.
4. The annoying random humming seemed too much for him to handle.
5. The garden smelled fragrant in summer.
6. Jane went to Norway last winter.
7. The baron came from Munich.
8. Never make a mean man mad.
9. Neal needs some lumber to build extensions.
10. Nancy knows that Mike might marry me.
11. Newton's comprehension of science knew no boundaries.
12. Mervin made a mess of the musical number.
13. Not under any circumstances can he be included as a member.
14. Nixon never ran again.
15. Mr. Morris met my neighbor Madeline in March.
16. Millie made lemon and lime marmalade.
17. Many men named Ned as a nominee.
18. Marsha and Mallory went to Macy's in New York.
19. That singing telegram made me angry.
20. A nasty note was sent to my neighbor anonymously.
21. Norman never sings in the morning or even at night.
22. Novocain numbs my mouth and tongue.
23. Diamonds make nice engagement rings.
24. *Mademoiselle* printed a column on anorexia nervosa.
25. Mike needed money to take Nancy on a romantic honeymoon in Miami.
26. Many men or women never learn knitting or needlework.
27. The man smiled with contentment when his team won the Indianapolis Five Hundred.
28. Don't smoke in the newly painted dining room.
29. Many men and women work in amusement parks such as Disneyland and Disneyworld.
30. My most memorable moment came when I sang with the Minneapolis Symphony.
31. Muriel will live in Merrillville near Adrienne Nowell's.

Paragraphs With Nasal Consonants

Most men and women make many decisions and one's friends may often be influential. Decisions made now may have major implications for many moons to come! Smart decisions are not made on impulse. Much information, not only emotion, is mandatory.

Marshall McLuhan maintained that the medium is the message. Many mass media managers market television time emphasizing the subliminal impact of commercial messages on teenagers.

Humor has significiant benefits. One man experienced pain in his joints and wondered, "If negative emotions bring negative chemical changes, might humor contribute to my treatment?" He programmed himself for optimum benefits, and noted increased pain-free time minus tension following sessions of merriment.

Muriel Montgomery married a minerologist named Emmanuel Glenn in Manila and moved around many times during her marriage to him. On one occasion, when residing in Arizona, Muriel became enamored of Indian customs and handicrafts. The museum in Phoenix presented a marvelous opportunity for Muriel to become immersed in many interesting readings and programs on Navajo Indians.

Rhonda Simonson came from an unfortunate family situation. It seemed that her parents never had time to spend at home, and were always running around town with friends. Consequently, dinner was never a family occasion and mostly consisted of weiners and canned or frozen entrees. Rhonda resented having to mind the small children and assume her parents' responsibilities. Her teenage years were miserable until she became determined to compensate for the emptiness in the home environment. She began to prepare nutritious meals for the family, related to the children more warmly and encouraged open communication during dinner times.

Words With Voiced Continuant Consonants
(suitable for improving oral-nasal resonance)

Words should be said slowly so that voicing may be prolonged throughout the entire word.

Monosyllabic		Multisyllabic	
new	rhyme	neon	loving
vine	loan	moving	movies
zoom	Mel	mellow	Molly
maze	loom	miser	muzzle
zing	mauve	mainly	zoning
thine	knees	nuzzling	venial
moan	zone	lion	leaning
kneels	noise	lonely	longing
mom	rain	morning	vision
man	ring	rolling	raisin
nose	worm	lemon	ozone
run	mine	million	alone
name	muse	immune	only
mine	aim	oozing	evening
hum	nose	numeral	manly
wing	wrong	Milan	mural
long	lung	muslin	minor
limb	maize	maneuver	manual
lamb	lime	mariner	menial
room	lame	Miami	millionaire
whim	vim	malaria	millinery
yam	whom	memorial	memorize
realm	elm	among	Amen
I've	knell	Emma	amuse
gnome	knoll	layman	mammal
known	nerve	Mimi	numbing
news	Nile	omen	Omar
noon	nor	rumor	amnesia
noun	none	amusing	alum
knave	Anne	memorize	annual
line	Verne	emery	vermilion
rhine	then	anomaly	alimony
than	vein	realism	living room
wane	whine	linoleum	aluminum
yawn	ram	Wilma	enamel
lean	lawn	naive	amazing

♦ *PRACTICE MATERIALS FOR FRONTAL TONE FOCUS*

Words Containing Front Vowels and Tongue-tip Consonants

To improve forward tone focus emphasizing tongue and lip movement. Useful for clients exhibiting cul-de-sac resonance, laryngeal hyperfunction, and limited mouth opening.

Monosyllabic			Multisyllabic		
neat	tip	net	lethal	chamois	shifty
knit	pat	nail	tipsy	shampoo	tennis
tab	tape	tea	patent	sheba	able
tail	deep	team	mitten	shiny	lady
tap	teal	knee	talent	babyish	Pepsi
teeth	lap	peat	bitten	demolish	tiptoe
thin	babe	bade	little	finish	taboo
tight	bad	bail	table	relish	tasty
cheat	bait	ban	tattoo	Danish	relish
chip	bat	bay	Lizzy	blemish	debate
laugh	bead	been	lowly	initial	tedious
tint	beet	bent	Lynette	beneficial	tally
tithe	bet	bib	pity	leadership	teddy
gnats	bill	bite	patter	tinsel	litter
feet	den	dam	batter	fiddle	teepee
sheath	date	dead	eighteen	chisel	petite
ship	deal	debt	belittle	chili	Betty
thieves	deed	deep	termite	achieve	Lilly
she'll	did	dip	petty	feature	tissue
shell	type	laid	battle	inches	British
shaft	lamb	lamp	city	moocher	fitted
shall	lane	lap	attention	peaches	latin
till	late	lead	Terrence	ditches	nineteen
fish	leap	tide	ballerina	chitchat	satan
leash	Lent	let	tablets	bleachers	title
flip	lid	light	nimble	busy	vital
fill	pad	line	peppers	fizzy	timidity
fifth	lip	lit	brittle	befit	lettuce
fib	paid	pail	bitters	Philippines	Teddy
chill	paint	peat	visited	fashion	aviation
tight	peal	peep	altimeter	differ	apple
teach	pep	pet	diameter	efface	tipped
tiff	pill	pipe	perimeter	jiffy	dainty
beach	pip	tape	nevertheless	infinity	thimble
cheese	cheap	sheen	lazily	pencil	athlete

Sentences Containing Front Vowels
and Tongue-Tip Consonants

1. "Tiptoe through the tulips," trilled Tiny Tim in falsetto.
2. We drank a pint of bitters and ate tasty tortillas, but Ted was a teetotaler.
3. Billy stuck ten tiny pins and needles in my voodoo doll.
4. Lynn and Liz raced to the sea to take a dip.
5. Write the letter on this white tablet.
6. Read the list of names to them at bedtime.
7. Their feet tapped the tiles as they danced to the band that night.
8. Sit in the seat at the left end of the little theater.
9. People vanish every day from city streets.
10. Terrence touched his front teeth lightly.
11. Lizards eat many little flies and gnats.
12. Linda prepares a tasty Bibb lettuce salad every day.
13. Penny needs an advance in salary to pay her bills.
14. Tea and sympathy help mend many ills.
15. Even if tired, Ted never buys tablets to help revive him.
16. Embarrassed people rarely interview easily anytime.
17. Betty made a beer batter bread with raisins in it and iced it with lemon essence.
18. Steve's dentist feels peanut brittle is sweeter than he needs and increases his cavities.
19. The stars in the Little Dipper light the heavens at night.
20. The Apache Indians stitched the skins into a nice teepee.
21. Neal appreciates that people feel differently in stressful situations.

Sentences Containing Voiced Continuant Consonants

1. The razor is always so noisy.
2. We run early Monday morning.
3. We'll all stroll home the long way.
4. He's as wise as an owl.
5. No one loves misery.
6. The royal family is rarely alone.
7. Mel loathes liver with onions.
8. No man is an island.
9. The lonely woman raises those roses.
10. I envision a long, lazy summer.
11. The man oiled the machinery every morning.
12. Will the sling harm my arm?
13. We will have more lemons than ever this year.
14. The sun shines warmly in summer.
15. Summer in London is lovely.
16. Mollie's new mother has a lovely home.
17. When he is lonely, we run over there in the morning.
18. The falling rain ran in waves along the railing.
19. Many luxurious yellow pillows were seen in their home.
20. Cinnamon was in misery when wearing his muzzle.

Activities to Practice Forward Projection

The clinician sits on the far side of the room and asks a group member a question. The group member turns to the next person and tells the answer at a conversational level. The group member then turns to the clinician and says the answer again using forward projection techniques (e.g., increased mouth opening, increased lip/tongue movement, and forward tone focus). This exercise contrasts conversational projection and distance projection strategies.

The student hums the tune of a favorite song, then hums a stanza alternating humming and saying the words of the song. The student makes sure the reverberation felt during humming is carried over into the words. Finally, the student hums first as a cue, then says all of the words of the song. If the tone focus is lost at any time, cue with a "hum" to regain it.

The student makes strings of /m/ words by changing one letter at a time. For example: mind, mild, mold, mole, mile, mill. The words are produced maximizing reverberation of the /m/ sounds.

The student thinks of favorite memories and uses appropriate projection, resonance, and the carrier phrase, "I mainly remember _____." Voiced continuants are emphasized.

Students in a group choose a country (e.g., France) and each group member, in turn, uses the carrier phrase, "I'm reminded of _____." A variation of this activity is for each person to choose a word in alphabetical order. For example:

"I'm reminded of Antoinne"
"I'm reminded of Bordeau"
"I'm reminded of croissants"

Voiced continuants and vowel sounds are emphasized.

The student relives a favorite moment, experience, or day and describes it. If projection is lost, other group members hiss softly to prompt the student who is speaking. It usually helps if the speaker stands across the room from the rest of the group.

The student imagines receiving $50,000 from a benefactor and discusses ways the money could be spent on the school. Appropriate tone focus must be maintained during the discussion. At the end of the discussion, the student summarizes the plans for use of the money, demonstrating projected speech techniques.

The student writes letters to famous people and reads them aloud, using appropriate tone focus during the reading.

The student counts aloud by sevens to 700, prolonging the voiced continuant /V/ sounds and maximizing frontal tone focus.

◆ PRACTICE MATERIALS TO ELIMINATE HARD GLOTTAL ATTACKS

Vowels in Initial Position in Words

Monosyllabic		Multisyllabic (First syllable stressed)	
arm	eat	oilskin	Oscar
own	ache	apple	angry
aunt	off	enter	over
act	old	exit	entrance
ice	oil	instant	enemy
ink	ox	operator	oodles
on	elk	open	eastern
oops	east	outward	ample
end	ear	outside	uncle
ax	of	obvious	anyone
each	out	everyone	unaware
itch	ease	utter	ugly
age	inch	ulcer	ultra
egg	ours	oboe	engine
odd	eight	oval	accident
edge	ash	ankle	angel
off	aisle	alcohol	alimony
ape	ale	altitude	igloo
aim	aid	olive	under
eel	up	edible	aardvark
oat	oak	alligator	afternoon
owl	ouch	artichoke	office
us	is	osteopath	amateur
in	eve	earthworm	outskirt
ooze	earn	afterthought	earthquake
and	oh	orchestra	orthodox
earth	oink	editor	oversight
oil	eye	auctioneer	optional
I've	ill	ice pick	ordinance
are	as	ape-man	islander
asp	ounce	icicle	oxygen
air	ache	Asian	oxidize
arch	add	eggshells	ex officio
oaf	I'll	opposite	officer
elf	aft	odious	emphasis
I'm	all	asking	embassy

Additional Practice Activities

The student identifies as many differences between hard and easy onsets as possible.

occur mainly on vowels
occur on stressed syllables
occur when there is too much effort or tension
neck feels tight
sounds like a grunt or click
feels jerky

The speech-language pathologist reads a word list and the student checks the words on which hard attacks occurred.

The student practices the transition from air flow to voicing in slow motion, prolonging a breathed sound and gradually adding smooth voicing.

/s/ ---------- /z/
/θ/ ---------- /ð/
/f/ ---------- /v/
/ʃ/ ---------- /ʒ/

The student makes a list of vowel sounds, practices producing the vowels preceded by an /h/, then produces the vowel sounds "thinking" the /h/ but not actually producing it.

The student practices word pairs:

whose	ooze		hit	it
hate	ate		heel	eel
he's	ease		hive	I've
hill	ill		his	is
ha	ah		how	ow
has	as		hoops	oops
heat	eat		hotter	otter
ham	am		high	I
hay	eh		hail	ale
hi	eye		heave	Eve
howl	owl		hash	ash

The speech-language pathologist questions and the student responds with the same answer each time, but varying vocal expressiveness. This activity involves practice of conversational timing and vocal and facial expressiveness, while the target response remains short. For example:

"oh"   "uh uh"
"always"
"I will/I won't"
"I do/I don't"

The student counts from 8 to 98 by 10s. This is tape recorded and then self-evaluated.

The students say names of people, states, cities, foods, or substances that start with vowel sounds. In a group situation, group members take turns and monitor each other's production.

The speech-language pathologist begins a sentence, such as, "I went to Alaska and I ate . . . ." and students repeat the carrier phrase and add items until each member has had a turn. The students repeat the entire sentence each turn. For example, "I went to Alaska and I ate avocados, eggs, oranges, artichokes, apples, and asparagus." Other progressive sentences such as "At Oxford I acquired . . ." and "In Iceland Eskimos argue over . . ." may be used.

Students share tricks used to facilitate easy onset. For example: elongating the vowel, linking the preceding consonant (e.g., "his answer"), "thinking" an /h/ before the word, saying the word softly, and breathing out on the word. After a discussion of various tricks, students read word lists and listeners try to guess the trick they were using.

The student has 5 minutes to construct practice sentences of words beginning with vowels and then read them aloud. Examples follow:

An ounce of ore equals and ounce of iron.
I am to exercise expertly all October in Ohio.
Our annual auction is always an exciting affair and attracts onlookers.
Ancient automobiles always act up in August.
Ann's Aunt Ursula exercises every evening in April.
Ellie asks for everyone's ideas and answers Anthea angrily afterwards.
Evelyn Ellis is always excited in autumn.

The student uses a dictionary to make paragraphs containing as many words as possible beginning with "ex."

The student thinks of words beginning with vowels as the speech-language pathologist reads the following list and writes the student's responses in blank spaces in a story. The student then reads the story aloud.

a plural noun _____
an adjective _____
a number _____
a verb (past tense) _____
a plural noun _____
an adjective _____
a verb (past tense) _____
a noun _____
a proper noun _____

Almost everyone is excited about art. Art is sometimes hung in
_____ and sometimes in _____ people's
    plural noun   adjective
homes. On occasions at art auctions, bids of _____ million
                                                      number
dollars, or even in excess of that amount, are offered. Once upon a time in
ancient civilizations art treasures were _____ in the
                                         verb, past tense
tombs of kings and queens. Our ancestors painted on the walls of
_____ . Many _____ carvings were made by
    plural noun   adjective
our ancestors. The value of art is often in the _____ of the
                                                noun
beholder. No two individuals always agree on everything and art is
not an exception. Although angels are _____ on the
                                         past tense verb
_____ of the Sistine Chapel, not everyone adores Michael-
    noun
angelo or even _____ .
          proper noun

Additional Sentences to Practice Easy Onset

1. Aaron asked for Amy's address.
2. In Alaska I observed interesting and unusual animals.
3. Emily is eating unflavored ice cream.
4. Andrew annihilated the annoying insect.
5. Aaron arranged exciting outings.
6. Obsequious people overpraise others.
7. Actually I am older than anyone else around.
8. The airplane en route to Israel arrived in Afghanistan at 8:00 in the evening.
9. Isabelle underestimates her own abilities.
10. Is anyone interested in investigating the accident?
11. Adam attends an auction every August.
12. Is anyone interested in another opinion?
13. Across the aisle Eddie ignored Annette.
14. Amy and Andrea are engaged in an angry argument.
15. Anthropologists are always interviewing Apache Indians.
16. Approximately 80 artists arrived early at the Australian Opera.
17. Understandably, Anna was appreciative of all your efforts.
18. The opposite of in is out.
19. Anne, Elizabeth, and Alice all entered the arena at 8 o'clock.
20. Everyone exhibited opposing ideas.
21. Isn't everyone educated enough in arithmetic?
22. I am interested in elementary education.
23. Imagination expresses an organism's inner ideas.
24. I am eating an apple an hour.
25. Eight egotistical egotists eagerly echoed their egotistical ecstasy.
26. Are any of you eating at Ellen's apartment?
27. Ask an instructor of economics about Eastern affairs.
28. Our annual auction is always an exciting affair.
29. Athletic activities are important elements on everyone's agenda.
30. In August I am attending a university orientation event.
31. Ordering oranges in an afternoon is an edible arrangement.
32. An ounce of ore equals an ounce of iron.
33. Ann's Aunt Ursula exercises everyday at an old exercise emporium.
34. All instructors of education are allotted an enormous amount of empathy.
35. Alice owes Ed about $80.00 and offered an I.O.U. instead.
36. Alice observed Andrea eating apples, oatmeal, eggs, and onions all at once.
37. Elizabeth's errors outweigh Eric's.
38. Evidently Ann's accounts are unbalanced.
39. Emily's anger over Adrienne's evil attitudes and actions is apparent in her eyes.
40. Albert's expectations are unreasonable.
41. Elliot's arithmetic is unsatisfactory.
42. Indians of Indiana are always undergoing every aid.
43. I always ask if all evidence is orderly.

44. Every iceberg acts icy.
45. If Agnew aches at apples, Edward eeks at eggs.
46. Edward entertains ingenues every evening at eight o'clock.
47. Any analysis of an active agent is utterly ostentatious.
48. An idiot accepts almost anything, even if it is incredibly unbelievable.
49. All irate adults insist upon alligators ingesting investigators of electrifying events.
50. An ardent admirer of Elizabeth admittedly inspected her assets.

Paragraphs to Practice Easy Onset

The amount of energy I am able to expend at any instance increases and decreases according to the environment around me. If, for instance, I am in a group of individuals with whom I am acquainted, the amount of available energy is enormous and I laugh and talk incessantly. If, in another instance, I am talking with an extremely close acquaintance alone, I am under no obligation to be extremely outgoing but am allowed to "undo myself," so to speak, and do as I please. The in-between amount of energy I expend is in a place where I sit quietly, as in class or when watching a television program. Then I am attentively alert, yet I talk more infrequently to others.

Almost 80 years ago, at age 18, my Uncle Ed traveled alone across the Atlantic Ocean and arrived in America. While on this excursion, he became engaged to my Aunt Edith, another immigrant from England. Their early years of marriage were not easy. Against Edith's intuition, Uncle Ed invested in the oil industry. Unfortunately, he lost his entire estate. They were forced to auction off all of their assets and start all over again. At this time, Uncle Ed announced that he intended to enlist in the army. Because of his ethnic origin, he was assigned as a special envoy to England. Edith accompanied him. They eventually returned to America in 1948 and ended up in Evanston, Illinois. In their older age, Edith enjoyed attending many social activities. Uncle Ed, still agile and active, spent every afternoon ambling about in the park, dressed in an overcoat and toting an umbrella.

Every afternoon at about 1:18, I experience an empty ache in my abdomen. I get anxious to eat an apple or an orange. In order to accomplish anything in the aftenoon, I must acquire only an apple or only an orange. Other appetizers I enjoy include apricots, artichokes, avocados, etc., but they do not appease the empty ache in the afternoon.

Edward Anderson accepted an invitation to accompany the ambassador of Afghanistan across the ocean to Eastern Asia. An extremely independent envoy, Edward embarked on an exciting adventure in India. After his arrival at the airport, he elected to amble around an unpopulated area. He approached an enormous amphitheater and exclaimed, "This is absolutely awesome!" Afterward, he enthusiastically accompanied the ambassador to the Afghanistan embassy where he was introduced to an assembly of Indian actresses and their escorts.

Amy Oliver, anchorwoman of the eight o'clock news, is only 18 years old. It all started in Arkansas when she was asked by Allen Osborn, owner of ABC News, to announce the entertainers involved in an Arthritis Telethon. Everyone expressed awe at Amy's ability. Ike Underwood was immediately attracted to Amy's emerald eyes. In a whisper, Ike asked Amy out, and Amy, of course was elated. You will be amazed to know that Ike has emerald eyes and was only 18 years old, too. Amy and Ike have remained together since that exciting evening. In fact, Amy Oliver will become Amy Underwood on August 18! They are both ecstatic!

On October 8, in the autumn, Ann Engle arrived in Oxford, Ohio, from Anchorage, Alaska. She entered into aerobic and acrobatic activities immediately. Unfortunately, she injured her ankle and it ached unbearably. She asked an orthopedic specialist for advice. He allayed her anxiety after examining her ankle. His expert opinion was for her to exert no effort for eight days before resuming exercise.

Paragraphs to Practice Replenishing Breaths

"I desire so to conduct the affairs of this administration that if at the end, when I come to lay down the reins of power, I have lost every other friend on earth, I shall at least have one friend left, and that friend shall be down inside of me." (Abraham Lincoln)

When I graduated from high school, located in Chestnut Hill, Massachusetts, I decided to take a summer off before I started college in the fall. My roommate, Tracy Donaldson, a very wonderful and close friend, asked me if I would like to spend the summer with her and her family in Lebanon, New Hampshire. Knowing how wonderful her family was and also, more importantly, how close Boston was to Lebanon, I decided to live with the Donaldson family. Why did I care about the proximity of Boston, you may ask? Well, I had a close group of friends, about 20 of us altogether, at high school, and since none of them were going on to college, they all decided to look for jobs in Boston. I, however, had decided to go to college in, of all places, Bloomington, Indiana, which is at least 1,500 miles away from Boston and all my friends. Knowing how much I was going to miss all of my friends in the years to come, I wanted to spend as much time with them as I possibly could, and the best way to do that was to live in Lebanon during the week and drive down to Boston every weekend, a short 2½ hour drive. Well, that is exactly what I did, and now that I am far away from all my friends, whenever I start to miss them, I just think of the wonderful times we shared while still in school, and also the times we shared during that wonderful summer in Lebanon, New Hampshire, and Boston, Massachusetts.

Allan and Bert May have owned the Apache Daycamp, located at 1600 Winding Brook Road, Hartford, Illinois, for approximately 17 years. The camp is actually composed of two divisions, one for children 3 to 5 years old, and one for children 5 to 14 years old. Approximately 200 to 300 children attend both divisions of the daycamp during the months of June through August each year. During the spring, both Allan and Bert May travel around high schools and colleges in the state of Illinois and interview male and female students who have applied to work as counselors at the Apache Daycamp during the summer. Most counselors are paid from $40 to $75 per week, plus room and board, and many enjoy the experience so much that they return for additional summers at the camp. Allan and Bret May supply transportation, which is usually in the form of a minibus, a large bus, or a van, and these vehicles are driven by the counselors who are 21 years old or older.

My little neighbor, Billy, the one with the red hair who always chases my dog around the block, has this annoying habit of collecting "treasures" from everyone's garbage cans and storing them in the bushes in my backyard. He is such a pest, and you wouldn't believe what he found on his last expedition and stashed amongst my rose bushes (the expensive ones I try so hard to maintain). He had been scrounging through the neighborhood, going from garbage can to garbage can, trash heap to trash heap, looking for something wonderful and valuable. Well, he found something, and it was something I did not want stored in my backyard, since I work very hard to keep my yard in good condition. I was looking out of my window, the large picture window in my living room, when I saw that little terror carrying something carefully tucked under his arm. It was black and furry and for a moment I thought it was a stray kitten, but I was horrified to see that it was my old fur hat, which I had thrown out when it hadn't sold in my garage sale last week!

Since time began, people have been fascinated by beautiful and visually exciting gemstones used for jewelry and adornment. In former centuries, precious stones were reserved for the ruling classes only, but nowadays, if one includes costume or fashion jewelry, gemstones are so numerous that it is hardly possible for the layperson to judge what is available. There is much to be learned about the formation, properties, deposits, manufacture, synthesis, and imitations of gemstones that it would take a lifetime of study to become expert in their categorization and description. The beauty of the stones and the appeal of brilliance and color do not always correlate exactly with monetary value. Individual's taste and preference vary, although knowledgeable collectors usually look for clarity and purity in gemstones as well as consider such factors as rarity, size, and cut. Some believe that as people age and feel the loss of their own beauty, they are increasingly drawn to collecting and wearing gemstones for adornment.

Some of the traditional symbols still seen today on dishes, furniture, tools, and barns were created by talented colonists who came from the Rhineland during the 1700s. The Pennsylvania Dutch colonists represented many religious groups. They developed a new way of life and a different style of art. Their folk-art motifs depicted flowers and birds and traditional symbols from their homeland. Their paintings, carvings, and textiles reflected their religious beliefs, their joy in their homes, and their pride in their craftsmanship. Pennsylvania Dutch homes were sturdy structures made of wood and stone and were extremely well kept, while the barns were built in the European tradition with oak beams and rafters. The women were wonderful cooks and contributed many recipes that have been incorporated into the culinary heritage of our country, the United States of America.

American colonial music was especially important to the early settlers, who did not have television as we do today, and the banjo was introduced to America by the slaves who brought their musical tradition from Africa. Many of the early colonists were religious people to whom hymn singing was an important part of their daily life, and wealthy families were influenced by European music and harpsicords, spinets, and violins were played by their children. New songs were created by the colonists as time passed, and the folk music of early America reflects the struggles of the new nation to describe the experiences of the colonists as they moved toward independence. As we listen to early American music, we are stirred by the tunes that soldiers marched to, that farmers hummed as they went about their daily work, and that women and children sang in the nursery, kitchen, and parlor. It helps us feel the everyday struggles in the new land, the happy optimistic spirit of the colonists, and the transformation of 13 young colonies into the United States of America, when we listen to the variety of music that characterized the emergence of the American spirit as we know it today.

Early explorers who thought they had found a western route to India named our native Americans "Indians." Early settlers from Europe, who were inexperienced in understanding how to use materials at hand, learned much from the native Americans who understood how to maintain the balance of nature, and colonists learned from them, for example, how to get sap from maple trees and how to plant pumpkins and squash. The colonists saw corn growing in the villages of the first Americans, and soon this crop became one of the most important to their survival in the new vast land. Corn could be eaten fresh or ground into meal, the husks could be braided into ropes and made into brooms and mattress stuffing, and in addition, dolls and ornaments could be made from corn husks. The early colonial families owed a great deal to the willingness of the native Americans to share their knowledge of how to make the best use of the materials available in their natural surroundings in the new land.

◆ *PRACTICE MATERIALS FOR VOCAL VARIETY*
IN PITCH, LOUDNESS, AND DURATION

Words to Stimulate Pitch Changes through
Meaning and Onomatopoeic Words

Definition: Onomatopoeic words — the naming of a thing or action by a vocal imitation of the sound associated with it. [Webster's Dictionary, 7th edition]

High Pitch	Low Pitch	Low Pitch
squeak	dungeon	boomed
creak	cave	sunk
teeny	deep	dump
peak	low	under
hiss	buzz	bummer
squealed	submerge	tomb
shrill	mellow	below
cheep	fruity	groan
yipped	thunder	moan
peep	doom	plunged
screech	thump	depths
tingle	thud	grave
rippling	murmur	humming
whistling	stroked	snore
snicker	plummeted	snarl
eek	tumbled	dreaming
tinkle	growled	sadly
surprise	grumbled	buried
chirp	shudder	gurgled
piercing	guzzled	slurp
twitter	gruff	burp
jingle	filthy	gloomy
trill	cascaded	dreary
soprano	dive	musty
piccolo	sank	rut
flitter	dud	fell
crest	delved	dropping

Contrastive Pairs

ping	pong		ceiling	floor
ding	dong		up	down
light	dark		smooth	rough
treble	bass		jump	hesitate
high	low		hissed	buzzed

Contrastive Pairs

hill	valley	fun	work
comedy	tragedy	minutes	hours
happy	sad	air	earth
delight	remorse	tinkled	crashed
flute	drum	top	bottom
sniff	snarl	bip	bop
piccolo	tuba	light	heavy
chatter	drawl	fly	elephant

Loud		Soft	
bang	howling	velvet	hush
roar	smash	feathery	muffled
crash	dash	mellow	peaceful
thunder	bash	tender	mist
slam	mash	silky	slumber
ouch	clash	tiptoe	coo
fire	bellowed	silent	delicate
clang	Stop!	soft	rustled
shattered	raucous	cloud	billowy
rumbled	shout	gentle	shushed
boom	explode	cuddly	swished
blast	noisy	fluffy	pastel
boisterous	brash	gauzy	furry
resounding	strident	quiet	souffle
blaring	deafening	soothe	whisper

Duration			
Fast		**Slow**	
tick/tock	halt	slithered	pull
blitz	galloped	pulled	blend
fleet	tap	strolling	molasses
flip	clap	stretch	creep
slam	shoot	linger	casually
pop	gushed	elongate	inched
flashed	swoop	trickled	leisurely
zip	snatch	oozed	snarl
zoom	wiggled	boring	sneer
whip	hurriedly	slowly	drawl

(continued)

Duration *(continued)*

Fast		Slow	
snort	knocked	slumber	languished
sniff	ran	murmur	waddled
sneeze	bounced	sustain	lazily
chatter	launched	wandering	sluggish
jabber	rushing	long	drizzle
lightning	gingerly	winding	dawdling
energetic	plucked	sleepily	doddery
plopped	grab	hesitate	marathon
suddenly	snap	prolonged	trudge
flitter/flutter	flicker	measured	dragged
accelerate	cracked	suffered	squeeze
bubbled	twitter	tardy	linger
babbled	catapult	waited	lulled
jump	splat	straining	languidly
immediately	hasty	poky	eternity
brisk	swift	plodding	lagging

Sentences to Facilitate Use of a Higher Pitch

1. The cook made a light, fluffy souffle that was airy and high.
2. He sang when he felt happy.
3. When we found out the news we were so thrilled!
4. She floated out onto the dance floor.
5. The pretty bird chirped and flitted about.
6. The effervescent champagne sparkled in the light.
7. Peter's eyes crinkled when he laughed.
8. In the high wind, the rafters creaked and squeaked.
9. Look at the star right up there.
10. We can see the balloon float right into the blue sky.
11. Did you see her climb to the very top of the ladder?
12. Did Jack and Jill climb the high hill?
13. His eyes twinkled and he said, "You're happy, too, aren't you?"
14. His parachute opened and jerked him upward.
15. Did you really think I'd do that?
16. On the night of the prom, Kitty was very excited.
17. As they looked up, the sky seemed filled with millions of stars, all twinkling.
18. She was at the pinnacle of happiness.
19. The politician's popularity rating shot up.
20. She climbed onward and upward, striving for the top.
21. The plane soared high above the clouds.
22. Is anyone interested in another opinion?
23. The tennis ball bounced over the net, then high into the air.
24. There was a tinkling sound fron the wind chimes.
25. I always have sweet dreams when I sleep with music.

Sentences to Facilitate Use of Lower Pitch

1. The submarine sank slowly to the bottom of the sea.
2. The miner went down to the depths of the earth.
3. The man crawled down into the deep, dark hole.
4. The mountaineer lost his footing and plummeted down to the valley.
5. I felt myself sinking down into a deep, deep sleep.
6. The parachutist jumped from the plane and floated slowly down to earth.
7. I sank deep into the plush velvet chair.
8. Grandfather spoke in a deep, gruff voice.
9. The prisoner was flung into a dank, dark hole in the dungeon.
10. I've been working and working all day and I'm so tired.
11. As we dug for gold, the hole got deeper and deeper.
12. The movie was interesting, but very sad at the end.
13. No one could have foreseen the terrible tragedy.
14. The *Titanic* sank to the bottom of the ocean.
15. The shark swam slowly in the murky depths.
16. Most people suffer from some depression.
17. The sun sank on the western horizon.
18. We delved into his deep, dark, and sordid background.
19. They toiled under the blazing sun.
20. The drums rolled mournfully following his death.
21. The mole tunneled away in the dark earth.
22. She stopped dead in her tracks when she spotted her old boyfriend.
23. My heart sank in despair.
24. We crawled along the bottom of the cavern.
25. We sat in awe as the soothsayer spoke.

Sentences Contrasting High and Low Pitch

1. The hang glider soared and then plunged into a down draft.
2. You take the low road and I'll take the high way.
3. Are you going to finish this, or do I have to?
4. She lifted her eyes upward to the sky, then down to the sleeping child in her arms.
5. The athletes stretched their arms upward, then bent down to touch their toes.
6. That woman sings soprano, but her husband sings bass.
7. As the men pulled down the rope, the boy was lifted into the air.
8. The kite soared up into the air, then landed with a thud.
9. After a long, hard climb, they suddenly reached the peak.
10. The party was great, but the morning after was a downer.
11. He scored a goal, but it was disallowed.
12. The low, dull drum roll accompanied the high-pitched, squeaky flute.
13. The fat, blobby snake slithered all the way up the tree to the very tip-top.
14. They enjoyed the picnic, but felt violently ill afterward.
15. "To be, or not to be. That is the question." (Shakespeare)
16. "If life is a bowl of cherries, how come I'm left with the pits?" (Erma Bombeck)
17. After a long, cold winter, tiny green leaves appeared on the trees.
18. I'm sorry, but can you repeat the question, please?
19. The young woman was happy and carefree until she received word of her father's accident.
20. Can you reach the top? I'm too short.
21. Don't get into a rut. Experience life! Live a little!
22. Will you help me please? I can't find it.
23. The boys swung higher and higher, but the rope broke and they fell to the ground.
24. The talented actress, at the peak of her career, became despondent and withdrawn.
25. He aimed for the last goal, but time had run out.
26. Those who reach for the stars never get bogged down in mediocrity.
27. Laugh and the world laughs with you, cry and you cry alone.
28. Tip your hat to Spring, and wave goodbye to Winter.
29. The trail climbs through the hills where the temperature is 40 degrees below zero.
30. The road twists upward and then plunges straight down.

Activities for Pitch Variation

Students ask questions of each other. The response is limited to "um hmm" but must be inflected in a variety of ways to reflect different meanings.

The days of the week are repeated with a different pitch level on each syllable. For example:

high pitch: Mon   Tues
low pitch: day   day

A variation of this activity is to require the student to generate multisyllabic words and speak each syllable on different pitches.

The student makes a statement and then adds a tag to convert the statement to a question. For example:

He's really crazy
He's really crazy, isn't he?

A variation of this activity is for the student to be given a list of different tags and then frame questions using those tags.

The student says a telephone number, using ascending or descending pitch levels in sequence. A variation of this exercise is to repeat the number, choosing various digits for inflectional emphasis. Students can also try to find as many different pitch inflections for their telephone numbers as possible.

The student generates as many pairs of "opposites" as possible and repeats the word pairs, contrasting the pitches. For example:

up   down
tall   short
over   under
overhead   underground

The student makes up sentences that have parenthetical clauses. The parenthetical clauses are information that is not central to the main idea and are spoken at a different pitch level. For example:

Bill, *he's my brother*, is a very good football player.
England, *where my relatives live*, has a lot of historic landmarks.

The student reads a passage aloud, beginning every second sentence on a lower (or higher) pitch.

The student reads a sentence aloud, stressing (with pitch variation) a different word on each successive reading. The student discusses how the meaning is changed and generates additional sentences. For example:

That woman insulted her boss after dinner.

Students think of a list of verbs that suggest motion and use them in senten- ces, varying pitch to suggest the motion. For example:

Eagles soar in the air
Leaves fall from the trees
The wind howled all night
The athlete jumped the barrier
The train lurched to a halt

The clinician presents a list of sentences to the group, and each student reads a sentence aloud. Then the student chooses an adjective to add to the sen- tence. On the second reading, the adjective is highlighted with an appropriate pitch change. Example: "The Christmas decorations were in all the shop win- dows." (Insert "sparkling")

Each student prepares a one-minute speech and presents it to the group. The goal is to use pitch variation to suggest meaning and feeling appropriately. A variation is to use pitch changes inappropriately and to discuss the incongruity, thus reviewing general rules for pitch usage. Example: "My most exciting day" and "Demons that visit me in the night."

"Feeling states" are written on slips of paper. Each student chooses one and then reads a short paragraph, reflecting the "feeling" in his or her voice. Other students identify the "feeling" from the vocal behaviors the student who is reading exhibited (e.g., envy, greed, malice, compassion, affection, sarcasm, bewilderment, excitement).

Students discuss vocal behaviors assoicated with a variety of roles and ages. They then practice simple sentences, attempting to create the appropriate vocal behavior (e.g., authority figures of different ages and professions, such as a young police cadet and an elderly police officer).

Sentences Contrasting Loud and Soft Volume

1. The music swelled to fill the room and then faded away to a solitary note.
2. The small, frail whimper grew into an anguished roar.
3. The children sat quietly in their seats until the school bell brought shouts of laughter.
4. The screams and cries of alarm sent everyone running, but the deaf old woman heard nothing.
5. The brothers argued in loud voices, but no one said a word when their mother walked in.
6. After the clamor and noise of the battle, there was an eerie silence in the field.
7. The bomb exploded, there was a moment's silence, and then the sirens began to wail.
8. The thunder rumbled and the lightning flashed violently; suddenly it was quiet and a rainbow appeared.
9. The girls were whispering across the room when the teacher suddenly slammed his book down on the desk.
10. The party was in full swing and the music was blaring; then John heard his parents' car in the driveway.

Sentences Contrasting Fast and Slow Rates

1. The hunter crept along quietly, aiming carefully, yet the sharp gunshot was unexpected.
2. She had waited patiently for hours, but the abrupt tap on her shoulder frightened her.
3. The voice on the phone droned on, but the click of the receiver brought sudden silence.
4. The thief crawled stealthily out the window, then took off down the street.
5. The runner slowly kept pace until the last lap, sprinted feverishly to the finish line, then collapsed from sheer exhaustion.
6. The leopard crept quietly through the grass, paused, then pounced on his prey.
7. My head was sinking into the pillow when suddenly I awoke, but soon I drifted back to sleep.
8. We stretched and pulled the taffy, then quickly snipped it into little pieces.
9. The stranger slowly stalked the scene of the crime, and then ran with amazing speed when the police chased him.
10. The race driver's car sped by the crowd and around the curve until it blew a tire and slid slower and slower to a halt.

Sentences Combining Pitch, Loudness, and Rate Changes

1. Each day is a grand adventure that ends with quiet sleep.
2. As your body races, keep your concentration still.
3. Love suffereth long and is kind.
4. Time can hang heavily, even as the minutes tick fast.
5. The rain felt soft but cold on her skin.
6. Sometimes anxiety can cause feelings of paralysis.
7. Whispering sweet nothings today, he would be hurling accusations tomorrow.
8. Some people who ride on an emotional roller coaster come to a grinding halt.
9. Tension and drama are sometimes used as substitutes for real intimacy.
10. An ardent Romeo wooed an impetuous Juliet.
11. She was exhausted by his restless energy.
12. Over the din of battle they could not even hear themselves speak.
13. Some laughed uproariously at the movie while others just waited it out.
14. Sometimes I fantasize about Europe while I do the dishes.
15. He wanted status and she wanted privacy.
16. The marriage of friends may be the funeral of friendship.
17. Violin strings can make beautiful music, but if drawn too tight, they snap.
18. My father had a quick temper, but he also had extraordinary courage.
19. The sun sank, showering the sand with a golden glow and sending a chill through the air.
20. As I stood in the sunset, I heard my grandmother's voice telling me stories I thought I had forgotten.
21. Susan saw him sizing her up and then smiling confidently at her.
22. In Alaska, chopping ice and hauling water is hard work.
23. Berries can be eaten on cereal or enjoyed one-by-one.
24. "To every thing there is a season, and a time to every purpose under the heaven: A time to be born, and a time to die; a time to plant, and a time to pluck up that which is planted." (Ecclesiastes 3:1–2)
25. Potatoes are nutritious and low in calories, but be careful about adding rich toppings.
26. Sleep through the night and you'll wake up refreshed.
27. The T.V. news blared as he picked at his frozen dinner.
28. A quick question should be given serious consideration at this time.
29. Building walls to protect yourself won't prevent you from getting hurt.
30. He was just passing through life, while she was enjoying every minute.
31. When someone says you have bats in the belfry, they imply you are crazy or weird.
32. "Life is mostly froth and bubble, but two things stand like stone: kindness in another's trouble and courage in your own." (Anonymous)
33. Pop it in the microwave and then savor it at leisure.

Paragraphs Combining Pitch, Loudness and Rate Changes

He hit the ball and it flew high, arching against the blue sky. The spectators looked up and squinted as they were dazzled by the bright sun. Then they gasped and groaned as the ball suddenly fell to the ground, out of bounds. The excitement, so intense a minute before, evaporated. The game was over and done. Victory had been snatched from the home team.

Sam was zipping along the freeway at 90 miles an hour and weaving in and out of the traffic. The top of his convertible was down and he felt the air whiz by his face and blow his hair. Then, ahead, he caught sight of a police car. He squeezed his foot down hard on the brakes and watched as the speedometer needle dropped back — 80 — 70 — 60 — 50 .... It seemed now as if he was merely crawling along the ribbon of road under the hot California sun. There was no exhilarating breeze to cool his face and body, and he felt as if he was hardly moving.

A mighty herd of elephants was ponderously grazing under the hot sun on that open plain. They lumbered slowly in the intense noonday heat, a slow mountainous group of flesh on padded feet. A bull raised his head and listened. A shiver raced through the herd and suddenly they were off, thundering faster and faster across the open plain, stirring a huge storm of dust in their wake, until they were a blur on the horizon. Then all was quiet on the plain again.

The assassin, dressed in black, slipped through the doorway into the dark night. He moved stealthily and made no sound at all. Everyone in the command post slept peacefully. High in the watchtower, a beam of light raced across the night sky. Suddenly a fuse was lit. There was a hiss as it ignited, and then a red line snaked through the blackness. A shriek penetrated the night, a high piercing wail of terror. Then the crack of an explosion as fire and smoke spewed into the air, and the building blew asunder with a deafening roar.

The band played jaunty tunes as the members marched across the green grass. Balloons danced in the air overhead, and a few white wisps of cloud dotted the blue sky. Spectators lounged on the side of the field, a few babies wailed in their strollers, and the hot dog vendors did a lot of business. The mayor mopped his brow, huffing and puffing with importance as he ascended the platform, and cleared his throat to begin his opening remarks.

Jayne was home late. She quietly turned her key in the door, gently opened it, and tiptoed up the stairs, her heart in her mouth. There was no light under her parents' bedroom door. She prayed the stairs would not creak. She could hear the dull thudding of her heart in the stillness. Then something brushed against her leg, and she gasped in fright — but it was just the cat. She was almost to the top if the stairs when she heard her father's voice, "Is that you, Jayne?"

♦ PRACTICE MATERIALS USING SHORT, EASY UTTERANCES

Redundant Phrases

This activity is useful in a group when the length of the target utterance is to be limited to two words but where spontaneous production is desirable. A list of nouns is presented to the student, who is asked to make an adjective from each noun and then to repeat the adjective and noun as a phrase. Phrase production is evaluated.

Example: slime — "slimy slime;" ghoul — "ghoulish ghoul;"
actor — "acting actor."

Anagrams

One student suggests a multisyllable word and the other students break it down into as many small words as possible. At the end of 3 minutes, the students read their lists using appropriate vocal production.

Example: Photography — pot, path, pray, hot, hag, hop toy,
trophy, toga.

Alliteration

The students think of sentences in which each word begins with the same sound. Each group member adds words to the sentence. For example: "Zany Zelda xeroxed Zion's Zebras."

Associations

The students choose a general topic (e.g., music) and find suitable word associations related to it. A variation of this (at the sentence level) is to name as many musical titles as possible. Each group member can take turns and other members can evaluate appropriate vocal production. To increase the cognitive complexity of this activity, the associations can be alphabetized.

Another association activity is to ask a student to think of something that:

Is over fifty years old
Juice is derived from
Has angles
Comes in a pump dispenser
Is made from synthetic material
Originates in Asia
Is a trademark
Is an amphibian
The student responds, "An example is _____."

Cumulative Sentence

One group member begins a sentence. The other members progressively add information. For example:

The teacher
The teacher said
The teacher said no one
The teacher said no one passed
The teacher said no one passed the exam.

Chain Sentences

One student says a sentence. The next student must continue by beginning a new sentence with the last letter of the last word of the preceding statement. The sentences must contain a logical progression of ideas. The group effort is tape-recorded and replayed for evaluation of vocal behaviors.

Count Your Blessings

Each student is asked to enumerate 12 blessings, one associated with each month of the year. A variation of this activity is to enumerate "pet peeves."

Famous People

Each student names famous people whose first and last names begin with the same letter (e.g., Alan Alda).

Each student names as many rock groups as possible and then pretends to be a disc jockey introducing each group in turn.

Opposing Proverbs

The clinician asks the student to state a proverb with an opposite meaning from the one the clinician quotes. For example, the clinician says, "Look before you leap" and the student volunteers, "He who hesitates is lost."

This activity may be used as a homework assignment or as a spontaneous group activity. It is hardest when students must think up the proverbs on their own. An easier version can be used by providing the students with a set of proverbs from which to choose. In this latter task, the activity becomes one of reading sentences.

An example of another activity involving proverbs is "scrambled sayings." For example:

Moss a stone gathers rolling no.
Nine a saves stitch in time.

Is saved a penny penny a earned.
Nose to your off spite your cut don't face.
Bush a bird the in the in worth hand is two.

Message on Answering Machine

The speech-language pathologist writes situations on index cards.
Students select an index card from a container and respond in 20 seconds or
less with a message to leave on an answering machine. The message must be
spoken in accordance with the student's vocal objectives. Situations
might include:

Call your parents' office and explain why you'll be late returing home
  from school
Call the vet to make an appointment for your cat
Call a friend to arrange driving plans for the ball game
Call your date and explain why you have to change your plans

Students must be sure to state their names, the date and time of the call,
and a succinct message.

Imaginary Auction

Give each student $20,000 in imaginary money. Inform the students that
once their money is spent they cannot bid any longer. Bidding opens on each
item at $200 and increments are $100 or multiples. The speech-language
pathologist is the auctioneer. Even though bidding may become spirited,
appropriate voice rules must be maintained throughout or bids will not be
acknowledged. Items to be "auctioned" might be selected from the following
list, or students could be encouraged to make their own lists.

Having the wardrobe of your choice for life
Having a lot of money
Having good health all through life
Being attractive to the opposite sex
Getting the very best education possible
Being famous

♦ PRACTICE MATERIALS USING LONG, COMPLEX UTTERANCES

Ten Years From Now...

Students prepare the sentence completion activity below as a homework assignment. At the group meeting, each student pretends to give an extemporaneous speech at a class reunion and presents a summary of what has occurred during the ten years since high school graduation. The other students monitor vocal behavior and provide written feedback.

In ten years my age will be _____ .
I'll be living in _____ .
I'll be the kind of friend who _____ .
One of my strengths that others admire will be _____ .
My future goals will be _____ .
My responsibilities will include _____ .
My most important personal possessions will be _____ .
The highlights of the last ten years will be _____ .

Rhyming Activity

This activity is useful for students who are working on vocal production at the sentence level. Increased complexity of processing is introduced while the length of utterance remains reasonably short.

A student thinks of two words that rhyme and announces one of the words by saying, "I'm thinking of a word that rhymes with foal." Other players ask questions by framing definitions. For example: "Is it a receptacle in which fruit is kept?" The student must guess the correct word from the definition (e.g., bowl) and answer in sentence form. The game continues until the correct word emerges. For example:

Statement: I'm thinking of a word that rhymes with foal.
Question: Is it a type of fuel?
Response: No, it is not coal.
Question: Is it a dark blemish on the skin?
Response: No, it is not a mole.
Question: Is it the spirit inside a person's body?
Response: Yes, it is soul.

"Ear Aches"

The name of this activity can be varied depending on the goal for the target response. For example, for students working to decrease hard glottal attacks, the target response "ear aches" can be used.

A student thinks of a word (preferably a common noun) and keeps it a secret from the other players, who ask simple questions to determine the secret word. In formulating each answer, the student must frame a response that includes the secret word, but substitutes "ear aches" for the secret word, with emphasis on the easy onset of phonation. Questioning continues until the players guess the secret word.

Example: (secret word = daffodil)
Question: What is the weather like today?
Answer: It is the kind of weather when there are ear aches.
Question: What did you do yesterday?
Answer: I gathered ear aches.
Question: Where do you live?
Answer: In a house with ear aches in the back garden.

Coffee Pots

This activity involves the choice of pairs of homophonic words. It is an effective group activity that can be used when students are practicing vocal targets in sentences with conversational timing and considerable cognitive complexity.

A student thinks of a pair of words that sound alike but are spelled differently, but does not reveal them to the group. Group members question the student, and the student must use answers that include one of the secret words. However, instead of saying the secret word, the words "coffee pots" are substituted and inflected. The activity continues until the word pair is guessed correctly.

Example: (stare/stair)
Question: What is your favorite sport?
Answer: I like coffee potting at people walking along the street.
Question: What did you do in school today?
Answer: I walked up a lot of coffee pots.
Question: When is your birthday?
Answer: Don't coffee pot at me when I tell you that it is tomorrow.
Question: Where do you live?
Answer: In a house with lots of coffee pots.

One-Minute Spontaneous Speeches

Students each choose a piece of paper on which a topic is written. Each student prepares an extemporaneous one-minute speech and presents it to the rest of the group. Sample topics follow:

Describe a character from a soap opera
Basketball greats
My dream wardrobe
My fantasy vacation
Tapes I couldn't live without
A nightmare day

Decisions

The speech-language pathologist presents students with a list of ways in which decisions can be dealt with:

Allowing others to decide
Putting off the decision
Drawing straws to decide alternatives
Not deciding at all
Impulsive, arbitrary choosing
Making a list of pros and cons
Evaluating and researching a number of alternative solutions

Students are then asked to generate examples of situations to illustrate the various approaches. They discuss the advantages, disadvantages, and possible consequences of each method.

The speech-language pathologist introduces the idea that "mistakes" are often the result of inappropriate decision-making strategies. Students are asked to consider the task of buying a car and discuss how the outcome is influenced by the following:

Personal values
Time available
Money (e.g., initial outlay, maintenance costs, insurance, cost per mile to run)
Significant others involved
Consideration of all options (e.g., new, used)

Topics for Spontaneous Speech Tasks
of at Least Three-Minutes' Duration

1. You can get good jobs without finishing high school.
2. A person who decides not to have children is selfish.
3. Girls should help pay on dates.
4. Fathers should feed, diaper, and bathe babies.
5. Life is a game of chance, so why plan.
6. Having a baby is a good way to get attention.
7. Men can make good nurses, flight attendants, and secretaries.
8. Life was much better before the Women's Liberation Movement.
9. There are some jobs that should be left to men.
10. It's a man's duty to provide financially for the family.
11. It's wrong to have sex if you are not married.
12. "A woman's place is in the home."
13. If you haven't had sex by your senior year, you're weird.
14. It's okay for a man to cry.

Formulating Solutions to Dilemmas

Students are given pieces of paper on which the speech-language pathologist has written short paragraphs describing certain problem situations. Students take turns presenting a dilemma to the group. The presenter is responsible for guiding discussion and reviewing alternatives.

Sample Dilemmas

Maria, in the eleventh grade, has a chance to get a job working for her uncle. She could have the job immediately and have her own money. The job is replacing the receptionist in her uncle's office for 6 months while the present receptionist is on maternity leave. She would have to drop out of school. What should she do?

Carol, age 15, is really attracted to Mario, who is on the football team. Mario has never paid her any attention and her friend says that she should ask him for a date. What should she do?

Ron is always being teased by his friends because of his squeaky voice. He avoids talking because of his embarrassment. The English teacher gives bonus points for oral reports in class. These are optional, but Ron badly needs to improve his grade by the end of the semester. However, he is afraid of making a fool of himself. What should he do?

Sean's girlfriend calls him a chicken because he won't smoke grass. Sean has poor eyesight and his optometrist told him drugs can affect people's eyes. However, he is afraid that his girlfriend will dump him if he continues to be a spoil sport at her friends' parties. What should he do?

Jeff has vocal nodules and has been told not to abuse his voice by yelling loudly. His father has a hearing problem and always gets irritated with Jeff and complains when he talks softly. Jeff hates fighting with his father but wants to get rid of the nodules. What should he do?

Diane talks a lot and is always amusing her friends with her impersonations and anecdotes. She is often hoarse because of the strain she puts on her voice. Although she knows she should be careful with her voice, she is afraid to give up her role as "life of the party." She thinks her friends will think she's dull and mousy if she isn't talkative. What should she do?

John's father is dying of cancer, but John doesn't want anyone at his school to know about it. He doesn't want people talking about his family or pitying him. Yesterday he got into a terrible fight with some of his best friends and acted very aggressively toward them. Now he feels bad and his friends aren't speaking to him. What should he do?

Megan finished a hard test and went to meet some friends at a fast food restaurant. She bought a shake and some french fries, and just as she was about to start eating, her two friends arrived. Neither ordered anything, but both proceeded to eat her fries. What should she do?

Standing Up for Yourself

The speech-language pathologist discusses the differences between assertiveness and aggressiveness. Students are asked to think of situations in which they find it difficult to stand up for themselves with family and friends. The speech-language pathologist then writes a list of strategies on a chart and asks students to apply them to the situations they've identified. Role playing may be used. Strategies might include:

Express feelings honestly
Offer solutions rather than complain
Respect others' rights
Criticize behavior, not persons
Take responsibility for own feelings
Verbally disagree without physical or verbal abuse
Gather facts before jumping to conclusions
Say "no" without feeling guilty

Rock Art

Have students select their favorite rock song, draw a picture to illustrate the song's lyrics, and then discuss the finished artwork.

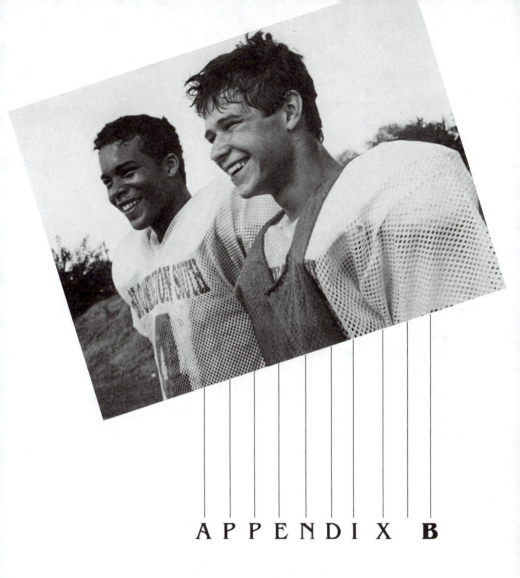

A P P E N D I X **B**

Practice Materials and Worksheets for Personal Growth and Awareness

♦ CONTENTS

◆ *PERSONAL HIGH-RISK INVENTORY*

This inventory can help a student identify the many factors relevant to a vocal pattern. It can also be used as a format for students to interview peers in a voice group and may be followed by a discussion. A variation, where the student interviews the speech-language pathologist, allows the speech-language pathologist to model responses and discuss individual differences in reactions to triggers.

Name: _____

Address: _____

Telephone #: _____

Check the following factors that you feel may affect your vocal condition:

Environmental Factors

Smoking _____

Alcohol _____

Noise Level _____

Dust in the air _____

Pollen _____

Recreational demands _____

Other (specify) _____

Health Factors

Eating disorders _____   PMS _____

Postnasal drip _____   Allergies _____

Throat clearing _____   Coughing _____

General fatigue _____   General tension _____

Sore throat _____   Aspirin _____

Illness _____   Other _____

Frequent upper respiratory infections _____

Use of antihistamines and decongestants _____

Inadequate energy release _____

Excessive mucus or dryness (specify) _____

Vocal Habits

Specific neck tension _____

Number of replenishing breaths _____

Shortened exhalations _____

Shallow breathing pattern _____

Specific laryngeal fatigue _____
Hard glottal attacks _____
Inappropriate pitch _____
Strained vocalizations _____
Excessive singing _____
Excessive shouting, talking, cheering _____
Limited vocal variety _____
Other _____

Personality

Afraid of silence _____
"On" all the time _____
Excitable _____
Nervous _____
Volatile _____
Depressed _____
Shy _____
Other _____

Comments:

♦ LIFESTYLE WORKSHEET

The amount of time spent in vocally challenging activities may affect an adolescent's motivation to change vocal behaviors. This worksheet focuses attention on the importance of time allotted to quiet versus vocally strenuous activities and can provide the basis for further discussion.

Instructions: Rank order areas of your life in terms of importance to you as an individual and amount of time spent (weekly).

Activities	Importance	Amount of Time
Television		
Sports (spectator)		
Sports (participant)		
Reading		
Religion/Church		
Family		
Clubs (specify)		
Paid work		
School		
Music		
Friends		
Movies		
Service to community		
Quiet time alone		

◆ *COMIC COLLAGE*

*Comic books often illustrate vocally abusive behaviors. In this activity,
students identify examples of abuse and list ways to avoid them. Alternate
strategies can further be explored through discussion and role playing.*

Examples of Vocal Abuse Cut from Comic Books	Ways to Avoid these Types of Abuse

♦ *INTERVIEWS ABOUT MY VOICE*

Through interviews, students can learn to discuss more openly the positive
and negative effects of their vocal behavior on others and gain insight into the
overall pattern of how they use their voices.

Myself	Brother or Sister
Positive: Negative:	Positive: Negative:
Teacher	**Friend**
Positive: Negative:	Positive: Negative:

◆ *VOICE IMAGE*

This activity stimulates insight and motivation. By providing practice in discussing their voices with the speech-language pathologist, students can define feelings about their vocal behavior and identify aspects of others' voices they admire and could emulate.

Things I like about my voice: _____

_____

Things I don't like about my voice: _____

_____

Things about my personalitity that can be identified from listening to my voice: _____

_____

People who have voices I admire: _____

_____

Pleasing aspects of admired voices: _____

_____

Which of these aspects do I possess? _____

_____

Which pleasing aspects could I acquire? _____

_____

♦ GESTURES AND EXPRESSIONS: ALTERNATIVES TO TALKING

Through discussion and role playing, students explore nonverbal expression as an adjunct and alternative to oral communication.

The speech-language pathologist writes the following words on index cards (one word per card):

rejection	nervousness	exhaustion
anger	fear	eagerness
disappointment	shyness	joy
surprise	determination	disgust

Students "draw" one of the cards and act out, through gesture and expression, the word on the card until other group members guess the word. Students discuss what additional gestures and expressions can be used, and in what situations these gestures and expressions can serve as alternatives to voice use. Then students role play, using both words and nonverbal communication, to convey the meaning.

♦ *REVISING ACCUSATORY STATEMENTS*

Sentence structure as well as vocal delivery can convey a negative message to the listener. By learning to revise accusatory statements, students become aware of how to constructively say what they mean.

The SLP provides a box containing slips of paper, each of which has an accusatory sentence written on it. For example:

You never call me.
Your room is a mess.
You won't have time, but I need help with my homework.
You're never going to take me to the game.
Don't yell at me.
That's a stupid idea.
You shouldn't do that.
Nobody here cares about me.
You always ignore what I say.
I just know you're going to stop dating me.
You're always lying.
You make me feel bad.

Each student must select a slip of paper, read the message aloud in an accusatory style, and then reword it. The revision must be worded to reflect the student's needs, feelings, or reactions. Beginning the statements with "I feel," "I need," or "I like" should be encouraged. Tone of voice and wording should reflect a positive, constructive attitude rather than an accusatory one. The group should be encouraged to discuss and evaluate the effects of the revisions. Characteristics such as loudness level, facial expression, and inflection should be noted.

◆ FAMILY "MESSAGES" ABOUT COMMUNICATION

All families and social groups have individual styles of communication. In this exercise, students analyze the direct and indirect messages inherent in communications between family members.

On index cards, the speech-language pathologist writes, "What does your family tell you, either in words or by actions, gestures, or facial expressions about . . . ?"

Tone of voice
Yelling through the house
Loudness level of stereo
Loudness level of TV
Dinner table conversation
Verbally sharing daily experiences

Cards are placed in a container and randomly drawn out for students to answer verbally or in written form. Sometimes there may be competing messages (i.e., say one thing, but behave in another way). Discuss these differences.

◆ ***LISTENING RESPONSES***

Whether listening responses are verbal or nonverbal, they convey important information. In this activity, the speech-language pathologist discusses the nature of communication as a two-way interaction. Students then list as many different kinds of listening responses as they can.

For example:

Telling an anecdote that tops the last one
Offering advice
Saying, "uh uh"
Frowning
Changing the subject
Being offended
Refusing to answer
Letting eyes wander
Asking questions for clarification
Interrupting before the speaker is finished
Talking to a friend while someone else is talking
Making a snide comment
Giggling
Complimenting the speaker
Saying, "I understand how you feel"
Saying, "It's stupid to feel that way"
Paraphrasing the meaning

Students pair off, and one tells a story while the other uses a particular listening response. At the end of one minute they discuss the effect the listener has on the speaker, then switch roles. At the end of 10 minutes, all students form one large group and evaluate and discuss the strategies used.

◆ *RANK THE VALUE OF INTERPERSONAL COMMUNICATION STRATEGIES*

By analyzing their own reactions to interpersonal communication strategies, students become more aware of the effectiveness of their own strategies. The speech-language pathologist can help facilitate emerging insights through questions or examples provided in the discussion. A student discussion leader can be appointed to prepare examples in advance of the session.

The clinician lists communication strategies (e.g., turn taking, question asking, active listening, affirming statements, advice giving, sarcasm, giggling, lying) and asks students to rank in order the strategies in terms of importance to them as listeners.

Discuss:

Which has the most important or least important value?

Which strategies have you not thought about before?

Does the value of certain strategies change in different situations?

Is complete honesty always possible? How can a speaker be honest and kind at the same time?

Can tone of voice help to make a negative statement more palatable to a listener? How?

How can a speaker's tone of voice de-value the effect of their words on their listeners?

Which communication strategies communicate respect for an individual who is being addressed? Does this increase their value? If so, how?

♦ *PREDICTING THE OUTCOME*

Every communication has some effect on others and on oneself. For example, control of one's behavior helps to make one feel good about oneself. This activity explores the outcomes of various strategies.

Have students predict possible outcomes of the following actions by writing the answers on a piece of paper.

Discuss.

> You scream and yell all the time
> You speak calmly even when upset
> Your eyes wander when you are talking to a person
> You maintain eye contact with your conversational partner
> You interrupt when you have something to say
> You allow others to finish speaking before talking yourself
> You usually do most of the talking
> You usually do most of the listening

◆ *SENTENCE COMPLETION*

When students are practicing short, spontaneous utterances, sentence completions provide a helpful structure. The sentences may be tape-recorded and then played back and evaluated. The initial portion of each sentence is read and the ending is spoken extemporaneously. The student may be encouraged to compare the vocal production during the sections involving both reading and speaking. For example, was the target vocal behavior maintained even during the part that was uttered spontaneously?

By next semester, I hope to have enough money to _____

_____ .

One thing I'd like to accomplish in school is to _____

_____ .

An evening of fun includes _____

_____ .

Something I'd like to try this semester is _____

_____ .

One habit I'd like to change now is _____

_____ .

When I have children, something I'd like to do is _____

_____ .

After school, the job I'd like to have is _____

_____ .

Some things I'd like to have accomplished in two years include _____

_____ .

My highest priorities in life are _____

_____ .

◆ *CAREER SKILLS IDENTIFICATION*

Many careers require a wide range of vocal skills. By tying vocal behavior to career objectives, the SLP can encourage greater motivation in some students. By first identifying those skills already possessed, the student may feel less overwhelmed by the effort involved in changing other aspects of his or her vocal behavior.

Identify students' vocation/career objectives on index cards (one career per card).

List vocal requirements of each vocation/career on individual index cards.

Identify those requirements the student currently possesses.

List those skills the student must acquire to be successful in each vocation or career.

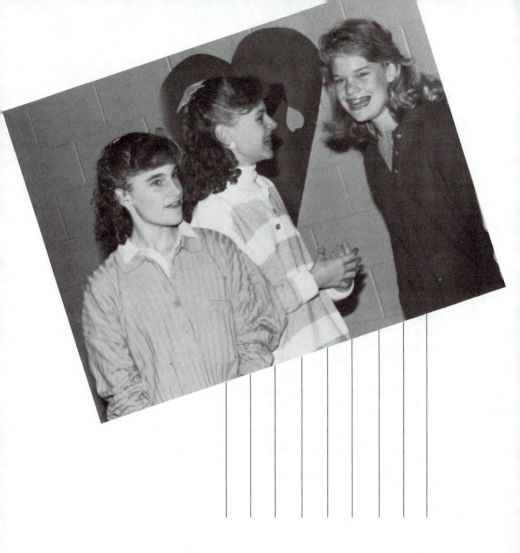

Subject Index